CARE AND CURE

T0143171

CARE AND CURE

An Introduction to Philosophy of Medicine

JACOB STEGENGA

THE UNIVERSITY OF CHICAGO PRESS

Chicago and London

The University of Chicago Press, Chicago 60637

The University of Chicago Press, Ltd., London

Published 2018

Printed in the United States of America

27 26 25 24 23 22 21 20 19 18   1 2 3 4 5

ISBN-13: 978-0-226-59081-3 (cloth)

ISBN-13: 978-0-226-59503-0 (paper)

ISBN-13: 978-0-226-59517-7 (e-book)

DOI: https://doi.org/10.7208/chicago/9780226595177.001.0001

Library of Congress Cataloging-in-Publication Data

Names: Stegenga, Jacob, author.

Title: Care and cure : an introduction to philosophy of medicine / Jacob Stegenga.

Description: Chicago : The University of Chicago Press, 2018. | Includes bibliographical references and index.

Identifiers: LCCN 2018020253 | ISBN 9780226590813 (cloth : alk. paper) | ISBN 9780226595030 (pbk. : alk. paper) | ISBN 9780226595177 (e-book)

Subjects: LCSH: Medicine—Philosophy. | Medicine—Methodology.

Classification: LCC R723 .S775 2018 | DDC 610.1—dc23

LC record available at https://lccn.loc.gov/2018020253

For Elah and Caeli

CONTENTS

ACKNOWLEDGMENTS

This book was written while I was at the University of Victoria and completed while at the University of Cambridge. Both universities provided ample time to devote to writing.

Though this book draws heavily on the scholarship of others, to keep the text readable I do not burden it with citations—the intellectual credit is noted in the Further Reading section of each chapter.

For close readings and detailed commentary on full drafts of this book, I thank Adrian Erasmus, Hamed Tabatabaei Ghomi, and Dasha Pruss. For comments on particular chapters I am also grateful to Susan Castro, Brendan Clarke, John Frye, and John Huss and his students. The undergraduate courses and graduate seminars that I have taught over the past several years suggested the need for this book, and much of its content started as teaching notes and classroom discussions. I am grateful to my students.

NOTE TO TEACHERS

This book can be used as a foundational text in an introductory philosophy of medicine course for students who have little or no background in philosophy. Supplemented with the additional readings listed at the end of each chapter, it can be used as a background text in an advanced philosophy of medicine seminar. This book is designed to form the core reading for such courses. Each chapter covers material for about one week of lectures or seminar discussions, and thus the fourteen chapters of the book can be used to structure a typical university course.

Sample syllabi for such courses are available on the dedicated book website (press.uchicago.edu/sites/stegenga/), and you can also find them on my Cambridge page (www.people.hps.cam.ac.uk/index/teaching-officers/stegenga). One syllabus is for a lower-level philosophy of medicine course, and another syllabus is for an upper-level philosophy course or graduate seminar.

This book can also be used in medical training as part of a course designed to elicit critical reflection among medical students about the foundations of their profession. Each of the four parts of the book could be suitable for particular modules in a medical curriculum.

At the end of each chapter I include further readings. Many of these readings are linked via the dedicated book website. I also include discussion questions at the end of each chapter that can be used to stimulate classroom discussion and to prompt student essays.

INTRODUCTION

Philosophy of medicine has become a vibrant intellectual landscape. This book is a map of that landscape.

Medicine is, of course, a hugely important practice in our society. Two of the main aims of medicine are *to care* and *to cure*. That sounds simple. But in the pursuit of these aims, medicine relies on concepts, theories, inferences, and policies that are complicated and controversial. This book describes some of these philosophical complications and controversies underlying medicine.

What makes a problem *philosophical*? This, unfortunately, is not a simple question. Indeed, it is itself a philosophical question. In this book I avoid heady debates about what counts as philosophy and adopt a pragmatic view: philosophical problems are those for which there exist multiple compelling and competing views, and which cannot be answered straightforwardly by empirical means. There are many problems like this in various domains of life, such as ethics, religion, and politics. A prominent subdiscipline of philosophy is philosophy of science, and philosophy of medicine is a relatively recent field of study within philosophy of science. Philosophy of science is the application of philosophical methods to science and the study of philosophical puzzles that arise within science. Philosophy of science usually addresses the epistemology, metaphysics, and logic of science, though it also addresses the history, sociology, and politics of science. Philosophy of medicine, in turn, is the study of epistemological, metaphysical, and logical aspects of medicine, with occasional forays into historical, sociological, and political aspects of medicine.

Each chapter in this book presents difficult puzzles about medicine and discusses and evaluates prominent positions on these puzzles. Does being healthy involve merely the absence of disease, or does being healthy require some other positive factors? Is a disease simply an abnormal physiological state, or is a disease a state that has an evaluative component? Is social anxiety disorder a genuine disease? What sort of evidence is required to justify causal inferences about the effectiveness of medical interventions? Is medicine good at achieving its aims of caring and curing—are most mainstream medical interventions effective? Is homeopathy effective? Does psychiatry aim to care for patients with mental illnesses, or rather does psychiatry aim to control feelings and behaviors that do not fit well with modern society? Should medical innovations be protected by patent, or should such innovations be contributions to the common good, unprotected by intellectual property laws?

Many of these questions are interrelated. For example, consider this seemingly straightforward question: are antidepressants effective for treating depression? Of course, this is in part an empirical question, and so answering the question requires a compelling view about what sort of evidence is required to answer such questions. Since that evidence comes out of a thorny social, legal, and financial nexus, a full understanding of an answer to this question requires insight into that nexus. Since antidepressants are said to target localized microphysiological entities, answering the question depends on a view about the relationship between the experiences of people— their feelings and behaviors and symptoms—and the activities of chemicals. Since the question is about a disease category that many people consider to be poorly understood and indeed controversial, properly understanding the question requires insight into the general nature of health and disease. These topics and more are discussed throughout the book, and insights from one part of the book help elucidate puzzles from other parts of the book.

Though this is an introduction to philosophy of medicine, this is not a book on medical ethics. There are already many fine introductions to medical ethics available. Rather, this book is about conceptual, metaphysical, epistemological, and political questions that arise in medicine. That said, positions on these questions have ethical implications, as you will see throughout this book. Although this is an introductory text, it surveys both the canonical core of philosophy of medicine and the discipline as it is now practiced by its leading researchers, at the cutting edge. The landscape has changed in the past fifteen years, and this book describes not just its archaeological substratum but also its current terrain.

Some very particular concerns in philosophy of science underly questions in philosophy of medicine. Classic topics in philosophy of science include the nature of explanation, the reality of scientific constructs, the demarcation of good science from bad science or pseudoscience, difficulties with inductive inference, and the role of values in science. Sometimes philosophers of science illustrate general philosophical problems with examples from medicine. For example, Semmelweis's discovery that the incidence of childbed fever could be minimized by careful hand sanitation in obstetrical clinics has been used to illustrate the importance of what philosophers call *inference to the best explanation*. No doubt inference to the best explanation plays a significant role in medicine, including diagnosis and causal inference. However, inference to the best explanation is foremost a general philosophical topic and not an issue specific to medicine. The focus of this book is predominantly on philosophical problems that arise specifically or frequently within medicine. Of course, many of the philosophical problems discussed in this book have more general import and arise in other domains. But in this book most of the focus is on philosophical problems that are central to medicine itself.

There are many ways to do philosophy. A philosophical approach I favor is sometimes called *analytic* because it involves the careful analysis of scientific ideas, using logic and expository clarity. Another philosophical approach I favor is sometimes called *naturalistic* because it appeals to facts about nature, gleaned from empirical science and the study of history. Much philosophy of science and medicine in recent years employs both approaches in a philosophical method that we could call *analytic naturalism*. This book predominantly employs analytic naturalism. However, to be a good philosopher one should draw on all the intellectual resources that one can, and so in places throughout the book I include discussions of other types of philosophical approaches to medicine.

Medicine is a vast enterprise. Clinical medicine is the familiar practice of physicians and other healthcare workers attempting to care for patients in a multitude of ways. Clinical research is the study of the efficacy of interventions, but of course medicine relies on more fundamental scientific research (sometimes called *bench science*) prior to testing interventions in humans. Medicine has many subspecialities, such as internal medicine, surgery, psychiatry, and epidemiology. Governmental policies and regulations control medicine. Medical research and clinical practice are guided by numerous intellectual and institutional movements, such as evidence-based medicine and personalized (or "precision") medicine. Philosophical problems arise in all of these aspects of the wide domain of medicine.

Since this book is meant as an introduction to philosophy of medicine, it has no unifying thesis. However, there is more to this book than a simple introduction to an exciting intellectual field. Precisely because this field is so young, distilling many of its salient problems into an accessible text has forced me to engage in novel philosophical work throughout the book. That said, I have striven to keep my own philosophical pretensions as silent as possible.

PART I

Concepts

1 : HEALTH

1.1 SUMMARY

Health is one of the primary concerns of medicine. Many philosophical accounts of health blur together analyses of the concept of health
with analyses of the concept of disease. However, it is useful to discuss the two concepts separately, though obviously there are significant connections between them. In this chapter we focus on health
and in the next chapter we focus on disease.

The concept of health can be analyzed on several dimensions.
Some people take health to be simply the absence of disease. Others
take health to be something more than merely the absence of disease, such as the ability to flourish in various respects. The former
view can be called *neutralism*, since being healthy on this view is a
neutral state, or a state of no disease. The latter view can be called
positive health, since being healthy on this view involves something
beyond mere freedom from disease.

Another important dimension to the concept of health is the role
of the patient in determining whether or not she is healthy. Some
people hold that it is only objective facts about a person that determine whether or not that person is healthy. Others hold that the way
a person feels about her state, regardless of objective facts about that
state, determines whether or not that person is healthy. The former
view is sometimes called *objectivism* because whether or not a person has a disease is supposed to be an objective fact about nature.
The latter view, in contrast, can be called *subjectivism* because it is the
subject's (that is, the patient's) assessment of her state that matters.

Finally, a related dimension to the concept of health is the role of
normative considerations in determining whether or not a state is
healthy. One view, called *naturalism*, holds that health is a state that
depends only on natural (biological or physical) facts. A competing
view, called *normativism*, holds that health is a state that depends on
evaluative (normative) considerations. This chapter describes these

various debates about the nature of health and assesses the leading positions about them.

There are various standards that philosophical accounts of concepts such as health and disease can employ. One standard is descriptive, which requires analyses of concepts to track various sorts of descriptive facts about a concept, such as the way the concept was used in history, or the way it is typically used today, or intuitions that we have about its proper usage. Another standard is prescriptive, which requires analyses of concepts to align with moral and political views about how we want the world to be and how we think the concept in question can contribute to this. Below we see how these two standards can reach different verdicts about an important concept like health.

1.2 NEUTRALISM AND NATURALISM

Health, according to neutralism, is simply the absence of disease. This is sometimes considered a "negative" conception of health, as opposed to a "positive" conception of health that holds that to be healthy one must have more than merely a body free of disease. If health is simply the absence of disease, then one might wonder what a disease is. The concept of disease is controversial—I leave the discussion of disease until chapter 2.

To articulate the negative conception of health associated with neutralism, consider its opposite. Here is one of the most prominent definitions of health, the positive definition of health written into the constitution of the World Health Organization: "Health is a state of complete physical, mental and social well-being and not merely the absence of disease or infirmity." Since this definition explicitly claims that health is not merely the absence of disease, it is non-neutral. It is a "positive" conception of health because it holds that there is something to health that goes beyond the neutral state of not having any diseases. A neutral conception of health denies this. Neutralism holds that to be healthy merely requires one not to have diseases.

To illustrate the difference between neutralism and a positive conception of health, consider two people, Lila and Elena. Neither has any diseases. But Lila grew up in a poor family, received a substandard primary education, and has few loving, supportive relationships, whereas Elena grew up in a well-off family, received an excellent primary education, and has many loving, supportive relationships. Lila ends up working in a physically taxing menial job where there are few people she can develop meaningful friendships with. She does not have time or energy to foster hobbies. Over the years Lila develops a bitterness toward her unfair circumstances and becomes hostile and unsocial. Elena, on the other hand, ends up working in a rewarding profession, meeting many interesting and friendly colleagues. Her increasing wealth affords her time and resources to foster playful and stimulating hobbies. Over the years Elena develops a deep satisfaction with her life.

Neutralism holds that Lila and Elena are equally healthy. Since neither of them has any diseases, and since neutralism holds that health is simply the absence of disease, both are healthy. Notice the appeal to well-being in the definition of health from the World Health Organization. If you think that Elena is healthier than Lila, in virtue of the fact that Elena's overall well-being is better than Lila's, then you might be drawn to a positive account of health. But if you think that they are equally healthy, because they are both disease-free, then you might be drawn to neutralism. Neutralism is closely aligned with another view about health, called *naturalism*.

Naturalism about health holds that health is a value-free concept. In other words, health, according to a naturalist, depends only on physical facts (or biological, or physiological, or any other natural facts). In order to accommodate mental health, some naturalists include psychological facts among those that are deemed pertinent to assessing whether or not a person is healthy. The most prominent naturalist account of health is Boorse's "biostatistical theory" of health, developed in the 1970s, in which naturalism is aligned with neutralism. To be healthy, on this account, is to have statistically normal biological functions: one's physiological parts and processes must operate with at least typical efficiency. A reference class must be specified in order to determine what typical efficiency is for a particular person, and on Boorse's account the appropriate reference class is a person's age group of a sex of a species. So, to assess the efficiency of my kidney I measure its ability to regulate electrolyte levels and remove organic waste from my blood, and I compare this with that of kidneys of other males in my age group.

Reference classes are necessary on this account because people have a wide variability in physiological functioning. Suppose Sara, an adult female, has normal levels of estrogen for an adult female. If Joe, an adult male, had the same estrogen level as Sara, then Joe would have dysfunctional physiology (and so would be diseased according to a naturalist account of disease—chapter 2). Similarly, if Mary is an infant female and had the same estrogen level as Sara, there would be a problem with Mary's physiological functioning. So to assess normal functioning, naturalism needs appropriate reference classes.

If we use inappropriate reference classes then we will make erroneous judgments of health. If we demarcate reference classes according to whether or not people are heavy alcohol consumers, then the normal range for liver functioning in this group will be worse than for nondrinkers. Suppose Ian is a heavy drinker, and we want to assess his health. If we compare the functioning of Ian's liver to that of other heavy drinkers, his liver functioning will appear normal. If we compare the functioning of Ian's liver to that of nondrinkers, his liver will appear to be dysfunctional. Determining whether Ian's liver functions with typical efficiency depends on the choice of reference class with which we compare the functioning of Ian's liver.

What makes a reference class appropriate? Recall that Boorse demarcated reference classes by sex and by age. What makes these factors appropriate for demarcating reference classes is that we know, on the basis of background theoretical considerations, that particular physiological functions differ depending on sex and age. But we also know, on those very same background theoretical considerations, that various physiological functions differ according to all sorts of features of different kinds of people. For example, we know that people with type 1 diabetes are unable to produce insulin, but it would be absurd to demarcate reference classes according to whether or not people have type 1 diabetes (one unacceptable consequence of such a demarcation would be that people with type 1 diabetes would automatically be deemed healthy because the efficiency of their pancreases at producing insulin would be compared with that of other people with type 1 diabetes). A standard problem that is raised for naturalistic accounts of health (and disease) is that nature itself does not demarcate groups of people into reference classes. Instead, we need to import background knowledge and evaluative content into determining the right reference classes to assess people's health. Thus, naturalism about health cannot be purely "natural."

The biostatistical theory of health is based on a notion of normal function, and thus, in addition to requiring reference classes to determine normality, it also requires an explication of the notion of function. We will leave this until chapter 2, where we study naturalism about disease (which is closely aligned to naturalism about health).

I noted that naturalism includes psychological facts as relevant to determining health. But at a fundamental level, most people hold that Cartesian dualism is untenable (this is the view that there are two distinct kinds of substances in the world: mental and physical). Most people are physicalists, who hold that the world is composed only of physical things. So talk of psychological facts is best understood as shorthand for physical facts that perhaps remain undiscovered. At first glance some aspects of medicine can seem committed to dualism—we'll see this in chapters 5 and 12.

1.3 WELL-BEING AND NORMATIVISM

Above I gave the definition of health from the World Health Organization as an illustration of a positive conception of health. A positive account of health, as opposed to neutralism, holds that to be healthy involves more than merely being free of diseases. Being healthy, on this account, requires the possession of various capacities, such as the ability to enjoy physically active endeavors and the ability to develop meaningful friendships. Of course, one's well-being is usually mitigated if one has a terrible disease, such as cystic fibrosis, and so absence of disease is an important (though neither necessary nor sufficient) component of one's well-being. A theory of positive health holds that the concept of health is similar to the concept of well-being. How compelling is a theory of positive health? Should we be neutralists about health, or rather, should we hold a theory of positive health? Is health distinct from well-being?

Well-being is itself a tricky notion. There are several leading accounts of well-being. One theory of well-being holds that a person is doing well if they are able to achieve their goals. Another theory holds that a person is doing well if they have certain basic capacities. Yet another theory holds that a person is doing well if they feel satisfied with their state. Most theories of well-being, obviously, require more than mere absence of disease.

What is the relationship between health and well-being? Most people agree that health is intimately related to well-being. There are three ways in which health might relate to well-being. Health might promote well-being: for example, being healthy allows one to maintain stable employment, which itself promotes various aspects of well-being. Or, health might in part constitute well-being: for example, reducing the symptoms of a headache increases my health and also, at the same time, increases my well-being because being pain-free is in part constitutive of well-being. Or, health might just be a kind of well-being: this is suggested by the World Health Organization definition of health noted earlier. Which of these is correct?

The two first possibilities appear modest and are almost certainly true. We have very good reason to think that being healthy can cause improvements in well-being. Healthy people are more likely to have rewarding social relationships, maintain stable employment, and achieve other important life goals. On any conception of well-being (goal satisfaction, state satisfaction, or capacity maintenance, to name the dominant theories), health contributes to well-being.

Beyond this causal relation, at least sometimes health can partly constitute well-being. I might have the goal of being disease-free, in which case satisfaction of that goal simultaneously renders me healthy and, on the goal-satisfaction account of well-being, contributes to my well-being. But this constitutive relation between health and well-being is fragile. Suppose I have type 1 diabetes and thus suffer from a serious disease that mitigates my health, and yet I am able to satisfy all of my life goals; on the goal satisfaction account of well-being, then, my health suffers but my well-being does not. So it's probably not universally true that health partially constitutes well-being. But it is at least sometimes true.

What about the stronger possible relation between health and well-being? Is health simply a kind of well-being? This is what a positive theory of health seems to require and what neutralism about health denies.

Let's return to the story of Lila and Elena. Are they equally healthy, on the basis of the fact that neither has any diseases? Or is Elena healthier than Lila, on the basis of the fact that many aspects of Elena's life are superior to Lila's? As we saw in the previous section, neutralism holds that Elena and Lila are equally healthy. But on a positive account of health, Elena is healthier than Lila.

As noted above, a popular conception of positive health and well-being is based on goal satisfaction. On such an account, people are healthy to the extent that they are able to achieve their goals. Suppose a primary life ambition of both Elena and Lila is to become a successful writer—thanks to the way her life has gone Elena is able to achieve this goal while Lila is not, and so according to a positive conception of health, Elena is healthier than Lila. There are several problems with such a view. One is that people might have unrealistic goals. Suppose one of my goals is to be an Olympic marathon runner. Since I am not achieving this goal, the goal satisfaction account of positive health holds that I am unhealthy. Conversely, people might have trifling goals. Suppose a person's goal is merely to live another day. That person could suffer from severe physiological problems and yet readily achieve her goal, day after day, and thus be deemed healthy on this account.

How are we to referee between neutralism and positive health? One approach is to determine which view is more closely aligned with our intuitions and with our linguistic habits. This would be to hold the two conceptions to a descriptive standard: on such a standard, the best conception of health is that which more closely tracks the descriptive facts about our intuitions and linguistic practices. On this standard, neutralism is likely to fare better. Another approach is to determine which view is more closely aligned with the way we want society to be and the kinds of lives we hope for people. This would be to hold the two conceptions to a prescriptive standard: on such a standard, the best conception of health is that which more closely tracks one's prescriptive views about how society ought to function and what aspects of our lives are valuable. On this standard, a positive account of health is likely to fare better.

A challenge for a positive conception of health is that the value-laden goals associated with positive health might be better construed as issues that are pertinent to society at large, rather than specifically to medicine. Since health is supposed to be a central concept in medicine specifically, one might hold that we should restrict our evaluation of various conceptions of health to standards that appeal only to medical issues. (Of course, the term "health" is sometimes used in nonmedical contexts, as with phrases like "the health of the economy" or "a healthy relationship," but these extensions of this medical concept into nonmedical domains are metaphorical.) Elena might be better off than Lila, but the respects in which she is better off are nonmedical, since neither needs treatment from physicians. We might wish that Lila's life would go better in many respects, but—goes this response—there is no respect in which Lila's health could be better, since she has no diseases. The ways in which Lila's life could improve involve education, labor, and social issues, and not medical issues. Positive accounts of health overextend the domain in which the concept of health properly applies.

Notice that this challenge to positive accounts of health, however, relies on drawing a boundary around the medical domain. What justifies this boundary? Again, one could appeal to a descriptive standard and respond by saying that this is just how the domain of medicine is approximately delineated in society. However, this response appeals to a relatively arbitrary and historically contingent fact. Alternatively, one could appeal to a prescriptive standard and say that we want people's lives to go well, and if that involves harnessing medicine, all the better—this would motivate a positive account of health.

Health is a valuable state, according to normativism. Though this might strike you as a truism, it is important to note that the concept of health is intrinsically value-laden according to such an account.

Normativism can agree with naturalism to a certain extent, in that normativists can agree that health has something to do with normal biological functioning. But normativism makes the further claim that the reason normal biological functioning is important is either because health itself is intrinsically valuable or because health is a means to other valuable ends. This is related to the question about the relation between health and well-being, because well-being is obviously an evaluative notion, and thus positive accounts of health are typically normativist.

Normativism can resolve some of the problems with naturalism. Consider the reference class problem. A normativist can argue for the aptness of particular reference classes by appealing to social values. Suppose an old man, in his 80s, has erectile dysfunction. With what age group of men should this man be compared in order to determine whether his condition is unhealthy? All men? All men who have reached puberty? Men between the ages of 15 and 60? Men over the age of 60? Men over the age of 80? We saw above that naturalism does not have purely naturalistic resources to stipulate the appropriate reference class for determining whether this man is healthy or diseased. Normativism, on the other hand, has ways to argue for a particular reference class. One could argue that sex is valuable at any adult age, in which case the appropriate reference class ought to be all adult men. Or one could argue that the course of human development is such that an active sex life is valuable for some periods of an adult's life, but as one gets older there is value in sublimating one's sexuality and developing other ways of connecting to partners, including emotional and intellectual connections, in which case the appropriate reference class to assess this man's health ought to be, say, men over the age of 80. However such reasoning goes, a normativist is not stuck with purely naturalistic properties in determining reference classes. A normativist accepts that determining whether or not a person is healthy is thoroughly value-laden.

Critics of normativism, however, claim that it faces damning counter-examples. We already saw some challenges to normativism, above. Here is another. Suppose we compare the health and well-being of two people: Jack, who has only one kidney, and Jill, who has two kidneys. Naturalists argue that Jack's health is lower than Jill's, but his well-being is not influenced by having only a single kidney. If Jack's life and Jill's life are equivalent in all respects except their number of kidneys, then, claim naturalists, Jack's health is lower than Jill's but they have identical well-being. Thus health cannot be identical to well-being, and health cannot be an evaluative concept. Personally I do not find cases like this decisive, because the case as described is question-begging: it stipulates that Jack's health is lower than Jill's, but this is precisely what is under dispute between naturalists and normativists. Normativists could deny that Jill is healthier than Jack, despite Jack having only one kidney, on the grounds that their well-being is identical. If their well-being is identical, then Jack does not suffer anything in virtue of having only one kidney, and therefore (responds the normativist) their health is identical.

1.4 OBJECTIVISM AND SUBJECTIVISM

Whether or not a person is healthy, according to objectivism, depends only on objective facts about that person's state. Those facts could be about purely natural phenomena (facts about a person's physiological functioning, or facts about the functional efficiency of a person in relation to her environment, for example), in which case objectivism would be aligned with naturalism about health (discussed above). Indeed, objectivism about health is typically aligned with naturalism about health, as in Boorse's account of health.

Conversely, whether or not a person is healthy, according to subjectivism, depends on a person's self-assessment of their health. What matters, according to subjectivism, is how a person feels, and not what the physical state of the person is. Of course, one's physical state typically influences how one feels, but there is no universal or necessary connection between physical states and one's experience of those states.

The difference between subjectivism and objectivism is not about whether or not health is "subjective" in a constructed or pejorative sense or "objective" in a realistic or praiseworthy sense, but rather is about which perspective—the first-person perspective or the third-person perspective—should be taken into account when assessing one's health. In standard cases the two perspectives align, as when laboratory tests conclude that you have a bacterial infection in your ear and you report pain in your ear. The difference between the two perspectives arises in difficult cases, in which the two perspectives do not agree on the assessment of one's health. We'll consider a few difficult cases below.

Both subjectivism and objectivism can be associated with either neutralism or a positive account of health. For instance, a subjective neutralist conception of health would hold that a person is healthy if that person reports no experience of disease (that is, if they report no symptoms). A subjective positive account of health would hold that a person is healthy if that person reports that they have the requisite valuable attributes that go beyond mere freedom from disease, such as ability to function well in society and achieve one's basic goals. An objective neutralist conception of health would hold that a person is healthy if their actual physiological functioning is normal, regardless of whether or not the person feels healthy. An objective positive account of health would hold that a person is healthy if that person in fact has the requisite valuable attributes that go beyond mere freedom from disease.

Here is a puzzle about objectivism. A person can feel fine and live a long and happy life, yet have a biological abnormality that they never notice. For example, many people have tumors growing inside them that are abnormal. Some of these tumors could metastasize and threaten other parts of one's body, but many such tumors remain benign. Because there is something wrong with the physiological state of such people, objectivism holds that they are not healthy. Yet, such people feel perfectly fine and may live a long life and die of natural causes unrelated to the biological abnormality. It seems odd to say that such people are unhealthy, and since objectivism says just that, this is a mark against objectivism. A concrete example of this is prostate cancer: the majority of older men have prostate cancer growing inside them, but few have any idea that this is the case, because the cancer does not cause any symptoms (medical scientists learn about the frequency of benign, asymptomatic tumors by autopsy studies, in which people who die of other causes are dissected to see whether they have any pathophysiological features). Ask yourself: if a person has a physiological abnormality that is permanently asymptomatic, is that person healthy or not?

What seems to be missing in objectivism is a sensitivity to the subjective state of the person whose health is in question. A person with a benign tumor can feel perfectly fine. If it was their first-person, subjective state that determined whether or not they are healthy, then such a person would be deemed healthy. This problem relates to the practice of screening, which we will discuss in chapter 11: screening involves hunting for cases of pathophysiology in people who have no symptoms. According to objectivism about health, there is no problem with screening programs, because such programs are simply looking for pathophysiology, whether or not a person is presently harmed by their pathophysiology; on the other hand, according to subjectivism about health, screening programs are problematic, because such programs amount to hunting for diseases among people who are, by definition, presently healthy (and even for people with benign forms of pathophysiology, most such people will never be harmed by it).

Here is an example that pulls in the opposite direction of the example of asymptomatic tumors. Consider a zen monk who gives up everything to meditate for the rest of his life in a cave high in the mountains. He is calorie-deficient, yet he does not feel hungry; he is exposed to dangerously low temperatures, yet he does not feel cold; he gets no exercise, yet he is not restless. This zen monk appears unhealthy, from a third-person perspective, yet in his own mind he is in a state of perfect ataraxia, serene and satisfied. From his subjective perspective this monk is fine. Is this monk healthy or not? Subjectivism says yes. Objectivism says no. Your intuition about this example might guide you to one view over another on the general question of subjectivism versus objectivism about health.

A basic challenge to subjectivism asks: why should we think that an individual has privileged access to their state of health? Most people are extremely bad at judging themselves, about many things in life. Consider an example from outside medicine. The Dunning-Kruger effect is the phenomenon in which people with low skills at a particular task estimate their skills to be better than they actually are, and conversely, people with high skills underestimate their skills. The psychologists Dunning and Kruger gave undergraduate students various tests in logical reasoning and grammar, and then the students were told to estimate their rank compared with other students—talented students underestimated their rank and untalented students overestimated their rank. So if people are bad at judging their skills on basic intellectual tasks, why should we think that people are good at judging their health?

A subjectivist could respond to this argument by noting that the analogy to the Dunning-Kruger effect is question-begging. A person's rank on an intellectual task, relative to other people, is an objective fact about the world. But whether or not a person's health is an objective fact about the world is precisely what is under dispute between objectivists and subjectivists. According to subjectivists, a person's subjective state is definitive of their health.

The debate between objectivists and subjectivists about health is closely related to the debate between naturalists and normativists about health, though we should not conflate objectivism with naturalism (and vice versa) or subjectivism with normativism (and vice versa). Objectivism and subjectivism are about the perspective from which a person's health ought to be assessed, whereas naturalism and normativism are about the actual facts that determine one's health. To see that these are distinct, consider the possibility of a position about health that combines objectivism with normativism. This position would hold that health is a state that is valuable to a person or brings value to a person, but that whether or not a state in fact does this is to be assessed from a third-person perspective.

Phenomenology is a different approach to the philosophical study of health and disease, which holds that we should consider the first-person lived experience of health and disease. Medical theory and practice stress the third-person perspective, and so, claims phenomenology, the first-person perspective should be reemphasized. Phenomenology is, then, a version of subjectivism about health and disease. We'll return to phenomenology in chapter 2.

FURTHER READING

Neutralism: Hausman (2015)

Positive health and well-being: Nordenfeldt (1987), Alexandrova (forthcoming)

Naturalism: Boorse (1977), Kingma (2007)

Normativism: Cooper (2002)

DISCUSSION QUESTIONS

1. Are health and well-being distinct concepts?
2. Consider Lila and Elena from §1.2. Is Elena healthier than Lila?
3. Is there a way to draw a principled line between treatment of diseases and enhancement of normal functioning?
4. Consider the zen monk in §1.4. Is he healthy?

2 : DISEASE

2.1 SUMMARY

What is a disease? This foundational question dominated philosophy of medicine for a generation. It is an important question, because controversies about particular disease categories can depend on assumptions about the general nature of disease. Such controversies, in turn, can have significant practical consequences—for instance, whether or not a health insurance program agrees to pay for treatment of a particular condition can depend on whether or not that condition is thought to be a genuine disease.

For example, is social anxiety disorder a genuine disease, or is it better to think of it as a social malaise? Is there a difference? Or consider another example: addiction. Is addiction a disease? On the one hand it seems compelling to think of addiction as a legitimate disease. On the other hand, addiction seems to be a problem with poor self-control. What about states that are precursors to actual diseases, such as high blood pressure? Are these pre-disease states themselves diseases? These are some examples of controversial diseases, which we explore in chapter 6. But to address these controversies with care we need to have a deeper understanding of what it means for a condition to be a disease more generally.

There are two main positions on what a disease is, and two important alternatives to these positions. One prominent account of disease, called *naturalism*, holds that diseases are simply dysfunctioning physiological systems (this is the flip side of naturalism about health). Another prominent account of disease, called *normativism*, holds that diseases are disvalued states (this is the flip side of normativism about health). An alternative to these two main positions, called *hybridism*, is a midway position between naturalism and normativism, and holds that diseases are dysfunctioning physiological systems that bring harm to those with the dysfunction. Another alternative, called *eliminativism*, holds that medicine can get by without a general theory of disease.

These views are conceptions of disease—they are theories about what disease *is*, or what features a condition must have in order for that condition to be properly deemed a disease. These views are not articulations of the experience of suffering from disease. To approach the latter subject, at the end of this chapter we turn from the conceptual analysis of disease to the phenomenological study of disease and illness.

It is helpful to distinguish the physiological basis of disease from the symptoms of the disease. When one refers to a disease, one might have in mind both the physiological basis of a disease and its symptoms (the total disease entity), the physiological basis alone, or the symptoms alone. Keeping this clear will help.

2.2 NATURALISM

In chapter 1 we described naturalism and normativism about health. The corollaries of these views are naturalism and normativism about disease. A disease, according to naturalism, is a malfunctioning physiological system. The most prominent naturalist account of disease is based on Boorse's theory of health, discussed above. According to naturalism about health, the concept of health is to be understood in purely scientific terms, and similarly, disease is just a departure from health. In short, naturalism about disease is an attempt to conceive of diseases purely in naturalistic terms, without appealing to normative considerations.

Here is one way that Boorse characterized naturalism: a disease is "a type of internal state which is either an impairment of normal functional ability, i.e. a reduction of one or more functional abilities below typical efficiency, or a limitation on functional ability caused by environmental agents" (1977). To determine what "typical efficiency" is for a particular individual, scientists just have to examine other individuals of the same species and demographic group. People in this group will have some natural variability in the relevant functional ability, and people at the bottom end of the distribution of this functional ability are diseased. For this reason this account of disease is also called a *biostatistical* theory of disease.

For example, phenylketonuria is a genetic disease that involves a malfunctioning enzyme, phenylalanine hydroxylase. This enzyme normally metabolizes an amino acid, phenylalanine, from food. Without phenylalanine hydroxylase, phenylalanine builds up in the body to concentrations that quickly become toxic. Phenylketonuria can lead to cognitive disabilities and seizures. Most people have properly functioning phenylalanine hydroxylase; to use Boorse's formulation, phenylketonuria is caused by a physical condition that operates at far less than typical efficiency. Hence, phenylketonuria is a disease.

Let's consider a nuance for naturalism. Boorse's definition of disease is based on a notion of dysfunction. To understand what dysfunction means, we should start by understanding what normal function means. There are two main accounts of "function" in the philosophical literature. One account assigns functions to entities or processes of a system on the basis of the causal contributions that the entities or processes make to the capacities of that system. For example, the normal function of the beta cells of the pancreas is to produce insulin, which controls blood sugar levels and contributes to the metabolism of glucose (this account of functions is sometimes called *Cummins functions*, named after the philosopher who developed the idea). The other account of functions assigns functions to entities or processes on the basis of historical steps that led to those entities or processes (this account of functions is sometimes called *Wright functions*, also named after the philosopher who developed the idea). In biology and medicine the pertinent history to assess function is evolutionary history. Thus, to say that the function of beta cells is to produce insulin is to say that beta cells have been under selective pressure to produce insulin.

Naturalism about disease is, at first glance, an intuitive conception of disease. (It is sometimes also called *objectivism* about disease.) Prototypical diseases like phenylketonuria are good illustrations of naturalism. Although naturalism about disease can seem compelling, it faces a number of problems.

To claim that a biological entity is dysfunctional according to a Cummins account of function, we need to be able to say what the normal functioning in fact is, and this raises a reference class problem. We discussed a version of the reference class problem in the discussion of health in chapter 1. To say what normal functioning is, we have to determine the reference class within which we assess normality. A person's biological functioning could be compared with the functioning of all other people, or all people of the same sex, or all people of the same age category (the breadth of which would have to be determined), or all people of the same sex and age category, or all people who have experienced similar external stressors, and so on. Boorse states that the appropriate reference class is an age group of a sex in a species. But as we noted in chapter 1, appealing to the two features of sex and age, and only to these two features, is groundless. Why not, say, race, or income, or professional status?

On the other hand, to claim that a biological entity is dysfunctional according to a Wright account of function, there is a different sort of reference class problem: we need to determine what historical period is relevant for assessing normal functioning. Selective pressures can change over time. Should we assess normal function by appeal to the selective pressures that the entity or process faced when that entity or process first emerged? Or should we appeal to more recent selective pressures? Or current selective pressures? The verdicts on disease attribution might differ depending on one's temporal reference for assessing selective pressures. A slow running speed, for example, may have been selected against in pre-agricultural societies, but in modern society it is no longer selected against.

Another objection to naturalism about diseases is that it is inconsistent with historical disease attributions. An example that has been frequently discussed in this regard is homosexuality. Homosexuality was long considered to be a disease and was even codified as a disease by the Diagnostic and Statistical Manual (DSM), the bible of psychiatric disorders. Of course, now we do not consider homosexuality to be a disease, and the Diagnostic and Statistical Manual has purged homosexuality from its list of psychiatric diseases. What changed? Why was homosexuality once thought to be a disease and is no longer? Critics of naturalism note that what changed was not a discovery about the natural facts regarding homosexuality, but rather, it was our society's moral views about sexuality that changed. Thus, according to this line of criticism, naturalism does not adequately track the way that disease attributions have been made in history.

To this, though, a naturalist has a clear rejoinder: naturalism is a conceptual and prescriptive analysis of disease, rather than an attempt to develop a historically accurate description of the way particular conditions were in fact categorized as diseases. Indeed, naturalism shows precisely what was wrong with once thinking that homosexuality is a disease: homosexuality does not involve a reduction of functional efficiency of physiological parts or processes. (However, notice that if we base our account of dysfunction on evolutionary success, and we admit that homosexuality decreases reproductive fitness, then it follows that homosexuality should in fact be considered a disease. To avoid this strange conclusion we could rely on Cummins' account of functions.)

Here's another problem for naturalism. Many people, perhaps most of us, have some sort of biological dysfunction, yet we don't know it because that dysfunction does not cause symptoms. For example, as we saw in chapter 1, many elderly men have prostrate cancer, but most do not know this because in typical cases the cancer does not cause any symptoms; such men can live normal lives and die at a normal age of other causes. Alternatively, sometimes a physical condition causes harm only under particular environmental circumstances. Consider the example of phenylketonuria again. Suppose a person lacks phenylalanine hydroxylase, but they live in a culture in which phenylalanine is never consumed in their food. Thus, the person never experiences any symptoms of phenylketonuria and, indeed, lives his entire life never knowing about his enzyme deficiency. Is this person diseased?

Here is a related problem for naturalism, and one that motivates its main contender, normativism: the badness of particular physiological states is not determined by the physical features of those states alone. Naturalist theories of disease must explain why diseases are harmful, and critics claim that any basis of harm attribution will be value-laden. Mere departure from statistical normality is insufficient for a state to be deemed harmful. A redhead has a statistically abnormal physical trait, caused by a statistically abnormal genetic trait. Redheads develop the pigment eumelanin far below typical efficiency. But this does not make redheadedness a disease.

Naturalism has a response to this problem. On Boorse's account, it is not just any abnormal physiological trait that counts as a disease, but only those that mitigate a person's tendency to survive and reproduce. That is, Boorse relies on an evolutionary basis for determining which statistically abnormal physiological traits count as diseases. However, evolutionary biology does not specify natural traits for populations, and humans have many goals besides survival and reproduction. To place survival and reproduction at the foundation of disease attribution is to value survival and reproduction, and while survival and reproduction certainly are valuable in most contexts, they are not the only valuable ends.

One of the motivations for naturalism is the presupposition that in order to be properly scientific a concept should be value-free. The role of values in science is controversial, with some philosophers saying that scientific methods and concepts should be value-free and others saying that scientific concepts and methods are necessarily value-laden. Perhaps naturalists think that in order for diseases to be studied scientifically the concept of disease must be value-free. However, at least in principle, a value-laden concept can be studied using a value-free methodology (thereby preserving an aspect of scientific objectivity—see chapter 8). Suppose an object of scientific study also happens to be an object of moral concern, such as lying. Such an object can be studied in purely naturalistic ways even if the object happens to be of moral concern. For example, if a sociologist finds that 38% of people lie to their spouse, that finding can be the result of a purely naturalistic methodology, despite the fact that lying is a subject of moral concern. In short, this "value-free" motivation for naturalism is not compelling.

2.3 NORMATIVISM

To call a condition a disease, says normativism, is to hold that a person with that condition is harmed by it. It is the disvalue of a condition that makes it a disease, rather than mere biological facts about the condition, according to normativism.

There is something intuitive about normativism. Here's an analogy. In a garden there are some plants, and some are weeds. What makes a weed a weed, and not just some other plant? Nature does not label some plants as weeds and others as not weeds. So how do we determine which plants in a garden are weeds? A simple answer is this: weeds are those plants that are not wanted in the garden. Weeds are disvalued plants. Similarly, diseases are like weeds: diseases are disvalued physiological conditions.

Normativism about disease holds that the concept of disease is value-laden, and any particular attribution of a condition as a disease is in part constituted by an evaluative stance toward the condition. That is, when we claim that some condition is a disease, according to normativism, we are implicitly or explicitly saying that the condition is disvalued. In other words, we are claiming that the condition is not merely biologically unusual, but that the condition is bad for people who have the condition, or harms people with the condition. (Sometimes this theory of disease is called *constructivism*.)

Recall that a problem for naturalism is that it does not have the resources to explain the basis of harm attribution of diseases. Some statistically unusual conditions, like phenylketonuria, are diseases, while other statistically unusual conditions, like being over seven feet tall, are not diseases—the difference is that the former condition is harmful while the latter is not. But, just as in the garden analogy, nature alone does not determine which states are harmful and which are not. Rather, it is our own evaluation of those states that determines whether or not a condition is bad for a person.

There is a threat that the dispute between naturalism and normativism could be merely terminological. Boorse, the arch-naturalist, distinguishes between "disease" and "illness." As we saw above, a disease for Boorse is a biological state. Illnesses, on the other hand, are diseases that have "normative features." When a person is described as ill, that person is granted special privileges, such as being excused for missing an exam, or receiving a mitigated judicial punishment after being convicted of a crime. Illness is value-laden, according to Boorse, whereas disease is not. So when normativists refer to "disease," they might be simply referring to what Boorse calls "illness."

If so, the dispute would be rather boring. But this is not all there is to the dispute. To put the real dispute in Boorse's terms, normativists would argue that there are no diseases that are not illnesses—of course, they would not deny the biological facts that some conditions are more or less rare, and are correlated with or cause other biological states such as symptoms, but those conditions are only in the domain of medicine if they also cause harm.

Normativism about disease has this advantage over naturalism: it can explain the basis of harm of diseases. Consider again the example of redheadedness. A redhead has a statistically unusual physiological trait, but does not thereby have a disease, since her rare trait (her red hair) does not cause her harm. Red hair is not disvalued (or at least, it ought not be) and thus having this statistically unusual physiological feature does not amount to having a disease. Normativism can make sense of this.

Of course, many conditions are bad for people, but not all such conditions are diseases. Consider poverty. Poverty is a condition that is bad for a person, yet it is not a disease. Thus, normativism needs a way to distinguish bad states that are diseases, such as phenylketonuria, from bad states that are not diseases, such as poverty. A typical way that normativists make this distinction is to appeal to sociological facts about the sorts of conditions that are treated by physicians versus the sorts of conditions that are not typically treated by physicians. Poverty is not in the domain of medicine, whereas phenylketonuria is.

The trouble with making this distinction in this way is that physicians deal with some conditions that should not be thought of as diseases. Consider an unwanted pregnancy. An unwanted pregnancy is a disvalued condition that physicians often help to manage. But being a disvalued condition that is managed by a physician does not make an unwanted pregnancy a disease. So this way of distinguishing disvalued conditions as diseases is insufficient. Moreover, from a prescriptive stance, this way of distinguishing disvalued conditions as diseases is facile—it is a historical accident that physicians tend to intervene on some disvalued conditions and not others, and we ought not base a prescriptive analysis on a historical contingency. Thus, the main advantage that normativism has over naturalism turns out to be one of its main shortcomings: harm attribution expands far beyond the domain of conditions that we normally consider to be genuine diseases.

We noted that naturalism is sometimes faced with the charge that it cannot explain changes in disease attributions over time. The example used was homosexuality. For a long time homosexuality was considered a disease, and now it is not, and normativists like to say that what changed was not our scientific understanding of homosexuality but rather society's attitude toward homosexuality. Normativists have a ready explanation for cases like this, which they take to be an argument in their favor.

In chapters 6 and 12 we will examine controversial topics pertaining to particular disease attributions. For example, is attention deficit hyperactivity disorder a disease? What about addiction? Or high blood pressure? These examples of alleged diseases show how important it is to have a compelling general theory of disease. These examples also suggest that different values can lead to different views about whether or not a particular condition is a disease. For instance, an active and social child who likes to move a lot, play, and exercise, is seen by some as healthy, but from the perspective of a stressed schoolteacher, such a child could be seen as a nuisance. Whose values should matter when assessing whether or not a condition is a disease?

A normativist theory of disease must determine the source of values relevant to evaluating disease states. Where do these values come from? Is it the values of the patient who has the disease that matter? Or the values of the society that this particular patient happens to be in? Or the values of a third-party observer? Or the objectively correct values, whatever those are, assuming there are such things? Answers to all of these questions can have unpalatable consequences. For example, if one held that the pertinent values were those of the patient in question, then a person could have a horrible physiological dysfunction and yet not be diseased, if that person did not disvalue his condition. Of course, these sorts of problems face any domain in which value-laden concepts are important, such as law and politics.

We have seen pros and cons to both naturalism and normativism about disease. This suggests that perhaps a middle view could be compelling. Hybridism about disease takes an important element from each of naturalism and normativism. From naturalism, hybridism holds that a disease must involve abnormal physiological functioning. From normativism, hybridism holds that the abnormal physiological functioning must be disvalued in order for that condition to be deemed a disease.

We saw above that naturalism does not have the conceptual resources to distinguish statistically unusual biological conditions that are genuine diseases, like phenylketonuria, from statistically unusual biological conditions that are not diseases, like redheadedness. This challenge to naturalism amounts to claiming that mere biological abnormality is insufficient for a condition to be a disease. However, this challenge does not question the *necessity* of a biological aspect of disease.

We also saw above that normativism does not have the conceptual resources to distinguish conditions that harm people and that are genuine diseases, like type 1 diabetes, from conditions that harm people and that are not diseases, like poverty. This challenge to normativism amounts to claiming that the mere capacity of a condition to cause harm is insufficient for that condition to be a disease. However, this challenge does not question the *necessity* of a harm-causing aspect of disease.

Hybridism takes both of these lessons to heart. Thus, hybridism holds that there are two necessary conditions that a state must have in order for that state to be deemed a disease: the state must be an abnormal physiological feature that operates at less than typical efficiency, and the state must be disvalued or harmful.

Hybridism inherits some of the positive aspects of both naturalism and normativism. A commitment to a physiological basis of disease is consistent with linguistic practice, historical disease attribution, and widespread intuition. A commitment to a value-laden basis of disease explains why a disease is a bad thing to have and why health is valuable, and it resolves finer-grained problems with disease attribution, such as providing a resource for apt reference class demarcation.

Hybridism about disease has an additional advantage. Since hybridism holds that there are two fundamental bases for a condition to be deemed a disease—the condition must involve a biological abnormality and the condition must cause harm—a medical intervention can be deemed effective either if it targets the abnormal biological functioning of a disease and returns it to normal (or at least closer to normal), or if it mitigates the harm caused by a disease. This explains why medicine has two basic ambitions: *to care* and *to cure*: when an intervention mitigates harm then it provides some care, and when an intervention mitigates abnormal biological functioning then it goes some way toward cure (we explore this further in chapter 10).

On the other hand, hybridism also inherits some of the drawbacks of both naturalism and normativism. For example, a commitment to a value-laden basis of disease raises the problem noted for normativism regarding the proper source of values to be used in assessing whether or not some condition is a disease: is the assessment to be done by appealing to the values of the individual with the condition, or of society, or by reference to our best moral theory? Conversely, a commitment to a requirement that a disease be characterized by a statistically unusual biological state requires the determination of the appropriate reference class with which to assess normality.

Some of these issues, however, are less challenging for hybridism. Take the reference class problem for naturalism. This holds that reference classes are not determined in a purely natural way, and this is a problem for a theory of disease such as naturalism that holds that the concept of disease is purely natural. But this is less of a challenge for a theory of disease that does not hold the concept of disease to be purely natural: hybridism can appeal to normative considerations to set appropriate reference classes.

To see this, let's return to the example of erectile dysfunction. Suppose two men have erectile dysfunction; one of them is twenty years old and the other is eighty years old. I take it as intuitive that the twenty-year-old has a disease while the eighty-year-old does not have a disease. But in both cases, let's suppose that their condition harms them. Naturalism claims that we should assess the functioning of the twenty-year-old by comparing it with the functioning of other men around his age, and we should do the same to assess the functioning of the eighty-year-old. Thus, plausibly, the twenty-year-old will be deemed to have a disease while the eighty-year-old will not, which aligns with our pre-theoretic intuition. However, we already saw that naturalism does not have the conceptual resources to demarcate reference classes in a purely natural manner, and so naturalism delivers the intuitively correct verdict only by sneaking in a nonnatural demarcation of age groups (in this case, say, between young men and old men, with some arbitrary cut-off around, say, sixty). Hybridism, on the other hand, does not need to sneak in this age demarcation: it can explicitly appeal to social norms and values to maintain that when it comes to sexual function an incapacity in a twenty-year-old is abnormal while an incapacity in an eighty-year-old is normal.

Critics of hybridism might raise an objection to this line of reasoning. One might note that the eighty year old is in fact harmed by his condition, regardless of whether or not that condition is statistically frequent for his age group (this is a version of the "common disease" objection against naturalism). Since medicine has some capacity to help such people, we might as well help. It would be strange to hold that such a person is not diseased, since he is in a state that harms him, and that state does in fact have a physical basis. To this a hybridist could just bite the bullet and hold that the condition is a disease, after all.

2.5 ELIMINATIVISM

Some philosophers and physicians claim that medicine can get by perfectly well without a general theory of disease. This is eliminativism about disease. On this view we should stop looking for the right definition of disease, in part because such work is a needless distraction and is irrelevant to clinical work, and in part because of a deeper suspicion that the disease concept and particular disease categories do not reflect the underlying reality of nature.

Here's an analogy from Hesslow, one of the first philosophers to defend eliminativism. A person brings her car to the mechanic because it does not accelerate as fast as she would like it to. The mechanic replies that there is nothing wrong with car, it's just that the engine is tuned in a particular way. Hesslow suggests that it would be a useless debate if the car owner and the mechanic were to argue whether or not the car is defective. Instead, argues Hesslow, the car owner should just tell the mechanic that she would like the mechanic to tune the engine so that the car will accelerate faster. The analogy is supposed to be this: arguing about whether or not someone has a genuine disease, according to the right definition of *disease*, is like the car owner and the mechanic arguing about whether or not the car is defective.

At first glance the analogy seems compelling. However, there is an important detail left out of the analogy. Suppose the type of car is advertised and guaranteed as having the capacity to accelerate at a certain rate, yet this owner's car does not accelerate at that rate. The car is, in fact, defective with respect to the advertised and guaranteed standard. The owner can ask the mechanic to repair the car to that standard and to have the manufacturer of the car pay for the repair. In other words, there is an important practical consequence of using a standard of defectiveness. The same consideration applies to the concept of disease. The classification of a condition as a disease can have important economic and social consequences. For example, the decision (by an insurance company, individual, or government) to pay for a treatment of a particular physiological condition often depends on whether or not that condition is considered to be a genuine disease. Moreover, having a concept of disease is useful for medical education and for communication between physicians and patients.

Concepts, very generally, are tools to help us navigate and manage the world. One could agree with the eliminativist view that there is no natural division of biological conditions into "diseases" and "nondiseases" but nevertheless maintain the general view that concepts, including a disease concept, can be important tools. Eliminativism neglects the practical consequences that disease attribution can have.

Some physicians are eliminativists about disease. For example, the psychiatrist Nassir Ghaemi claims that one does not need a general theory of disease or specifically of mental illnesses in order to identify particular psychiatric diseases. This is not compelling. In general, to justify that some entity, x, is a member of a class of things X, one at least needs to know what sorts of things truly are members of X. To know this, we could simply stipulate class membership (for example: "all objects currently on my desk are members of X; x is currently on my desk; therefore, x is an X"), but this is not very useful for the scientific discovery of disease categories because disease categories should not be arbitrary or gerrymandered this way. Another way to know whether x is a member of a class of things X is to have a general theory about the things that make up X, and then to determine whether some particular entity x is like those things. In other words, to properly identify a particular condition as a disease, we could use a general theory of disease. This latter method of determining whether some condition is a disease is superior to the former method of mere stipulation.

2.6 PHENOMENOLOGY

The theories about disease that we've studied so far are concerned with the fundamental nature of disease. These positions are asking what disease *is*. Phenomenology asks a different, though related, question. Phenomenology asks: what is it like to be diseased?

Phenomenology is a philosophical approach that developed out of French and German philosophy in the early- to mid-twentieth century. Merleau-Ponty, Husserl, and Heidegger were important figures in this movement, and in recent years many scholars have applied the phenomenological approach to various aspects of medicine. Phenomenology is less analytic and prescriptive than the "analytic naturalist" approach taken in most of this book; rather, phenomenology aims to richly describe the experience of having a disease. Some phenomenologists distinguish between disease and illness: a disease, according to this approach, is a physical or biological disturbance of the body, while illness is the lived experience of that disturbance. With this distinction in place, phenomenologists focus on the latter and articulate many aspects of illness that can be neglected when one focuses only on biological aspects of disease.

This approach notes how being ill can change one's life and one's experience of life. Our capacity to get by in the world is hampered by an illness, and phenomenology aims to articulate this. For example, an illness could entail that you cannot leave the house, which in turn entails that your possibilities for socializing are mitigated—the illness affects your personal relationships, and this is not something that can be understood merely by describing the physical aspects of your disease.

A critic of phenomenology could say that medicine has always aimed to describe the symptoms of diseases, and since the lived experience of an illness is a symptom of a disease, phenomenology doesn't add much. On the other hand, precisely because phenomenology aims to very carefully articulate the first-person experience of illnesses, the approach can unearth features of disease and illness that medicine has thus far overlooked. For example, a phenomenological approach to depression suggests that depression involves deep feelings of guilt, which can shape the possibilities of other emotional experiences—with this account of depression in place, psychiatry can rethink what it means to be depressed.

FURTHER READING

Naturalism: Boorse (1977), Boorse (1997), Lemoine (2013)
Normativism: Cooper (2002), Engelhardt (1976), Carel (2013)
Hybridism: Horwitz and Wakefield (2007)
Eliminativism: Hesslow (1993), Ereshefsky (2009)
Phenomenology: Carel (2013), Ratcliffe (2010)

DISCUSSION QUESTIONS

1. What is a disease?
2. Do we need a general concept of disease?
3. If a condition does not cause symptoms, can that condition be a disease?
4. Give an example of a condition for which normativism and naturalism disagree about whether or not the condition is a disease. Which of these (normativism or naturalism) makes most sense of this condition?

3 : DEATH

Most of us fear death. What is this fearful event that happens to all of us? Is death bad? If so, how exactly is it bad? These questions may, at first, seem to have obvious answers. But upon reflection these questions turn out to be deeply perplexing.

Death is a central part of medicine. One aim of medicine is to intervene on diseases to avoid death. So a central assumption of medical practice is that death is something to be avoided. In many cases the avoidance of death comes at a great personal, financial, and institutional cost. Why should we strive so hard to avoid death? Is death so bad? In the end, we always fail at this ambition—we all die. For many of us death occurs in the context of medicine: consuming medications, or using life-support machines, to avoid death.

The famous American novelist Cormac McCarthy had one of his characters say "How surely are the dead beyond death. Death is what the living carry with them. A state of dread, like some uncanny foretaste of a bitter memory. But the dead do not remember and nothingness is not a curse." In other words, death is not something to fear. Is this right?

What is death? Most of us hold an untutored view that death involves the permanent cessation of biological functioning of an organism. There is surely something right about this. However, although the death of an organism is important in medicine, there is another kind of death that is important, namely, death of a person. Personhood is an important theoretical concept in our moral thinking. There are reasons to think that death of an organism may be sufficient for death of a person (though some argue against that), but there are reasons to think that death of an organism is not necessary for death of a person. This chapter explores this puzzling issue.

Having a well-grounded theoretical understanding of death gives us a more sophisticated way to think about the ethics of killing. Although it might sound strange to talk about killing in the context of medicine, we must think very carefully about the contexts in which abortion, euthanasia, and the withdrawal of life support are permitted. This chapter does not address these applied ethical questions head on (because they are best left for a book on medical ethics), but rather, this chapter focuses on the foundational issues on which such applied ethical questions are based.

3.2 DEFINING DEATH

Death, you might think, is merely the cessation of life. So when it comes to defining death, there is little to puzzle over: first we must figure out what life is, and then we simply define death as the state that holds after life has ceased. This is a fine start, but it misses much of what is important about death.

When defining what death is, one might be addressing two distinct, though related, questions. One question, which we could call the biology of death, is to ask what conditions are necessary or sufficient for an organism to be dead. To keep this question focused on medicine, it helps to constrain the question of death to humans, since it is reasonable to expect that the biological conditions of death for mammals are very different than the biological conditions of death for, say, mushrooms (though the biological conditions of death for such different species might be similar when described at a sufficiently abstract level). The conditions that constitute the death of an organism are *bodily* states. The biological death of a human might require the permanent cessation of the functioning of the heart (cardiac death), of the lungs (pulmonary death), of the entire brain (whole brain death), or of particular parts of the brain, such as the cortex (higher brain death).

The other question, which we could call the metaphysics of death, is to ask what conditions are necessary or sufficient for the loss of a person. Personhood is a theoretical concept that is embedded in our legal and moral thinking and practices. Compared with the death of an organism, it is less obvious what conditions constitute the death of a person. These conditions are not necessarily bodily states (though they might depend on bodily states)—religious perspectives might hold that the conditions that constitute the death of a person involve the loss of a *soul*, while a more secular perspective might hold that death of a person involves the loss of *consciousness*. The two questions are related, of course, because the metaphysical conditions of death might depend fundamentally on biological conditions.

Indeed, one position about the metaphysics of death is what we could call *eliminativism* (no pun intended). Death just *is* the loss of organismic functioning, according to metaphysical eliminativism about death. This position is eliminativist because it holds that there is no soul or consciousness or other nonbiological entities that are sometimes said to constitute a person, and thus the death of a person just is the death of the corresponding organism. A person is not composed of two kinds of things: biological properties and, say, soulful properties. This position is committed to a form of reductionism (see chapter 5), at least about mental properties. Biological activities like respiration, photosynthesis, cellular homeostasis, and digestion are necessary for an organism to live, and death of an organism is just the loss of life, according to this view. A problem with this view is that it neglects phenomenological evidence: we have experience of what it is like to be a person, with feelings and memories and self-reflective consciousness. The loss of *that* is what really matters when a person dies. Moreover, since personhood is such an important concept for moral theory and practice, the loss of the status of person is a crucially important event characterized by the most profound sort of loss an individual can experience. From a legal and moral perspective, that loss is death.

Many moral theorists take particular cognitive features, especially consciousness, to determine what sorts of entities in the world have rights and duties. Rights and duties arise insofar as we are *persons*; conversely, rights and duties do not exist merely in virtue of the fact that we are organisms. What is it about us as persons that generates these otherwise spooky nonphysical properties? One common answer is consciousness. It is our consciousness and other features of our complex cognitive functioning that set us apart from other animals and give us a particular moral status. Of course, our consciousness might arise purely as a result of biological properties, but it is the consciousness itself and not those biological properties that are of fundamental importance. This position is therefore opposed to eliminativism about death. We can call this position *death dualism*. That is because the position maintains that there are essentially two different kinds of death: death of the organism and death of the person. Death of the organism occurs when the relevant bodily processes cease to function. Death of the person occurs when the relevant moral-status-conferring processes cease to function. Death dualism does not necessarily assume substance dualism (the view made famous by Descartes, that there are two fundamental kinds of things in the world: physical and mental), because personhood might be (and almost certainly is) a result of physical entities and processes. Death dualism holds that the cessation of all physical functioning of an organism is sufficient for a person to die, but it is far from necessary.

Importantly, according to death dualism, death of the person might occur before death of the organism. For instance, if a person has permanently lost consciousness but maintains cardiac and pulmonary functioning, then, arguably, the organism is alive but the person is dead. Such patients are said to be in a "permanent vegetative state." We return to such cases in §3.4.

The question about the metaphysics of death is closely related to the question about the biology of death, even if the death of the person (a metaphysical event) does not simply reduce to the death of the organism (a biological event).

So, then, what are the biological conditions of death? By now it should be clear that this depends on whether or not one is asking about the death of an organism or the death of a person, and whether or not one's metaphysical view of death maintains that there is a real distinction between these two kinds of death. Let us suppose that there is such a distinction. The death of an organism occurs when there is an irreversible cessation of the physiological functioning required to keep the organism alive—for mammals it is standard to think that permanent cessation of cardiopulmonary functioning constitutes death of an organism. The death of a person occurs when there is an irreversible cessation of the capacity for personhood. But what is that? If one holds that consciousness is necessary and sufficient for personhood, then one will hold that permanent loss of consciousness is necessary and sufficient for the death of a person.

Consciousness is, of course, an extremely complex and poorly understood phenomenon. There are, though, some basic things about consciousness that neuroscience understands well enough. Consciousness is, in humans at least, a function of the brain, and specifically a function of particular regions of the brain, especially the cortex (consciousness may also involve other parts of the body, which is a thesis known as *embodied cognition*). Notice that all it takes for a person to permanently lose their capacity for consciousness is damage to higher brain processes that occur in specific regions like the cortex. According to the "higher brain death" definition of death, death of a person occurs when higher brain functioning permanently ceases.

In contrast, the "whole brain death" definition of death holds that death of a person occurs when the entire brain of that person ceases to function. Here is the definition of death according to the US President's Commission (1981), which is disjunctive: "an individual who has sustained either (1) irreversible cessation of circulatory and respiratory functions, or (2) irreversible cessation of all functions of the entire brain, including the brainstem, is dead." The second disjunct is the whole brain definition of death.

This is not merely an academic dispute. Remember that what is at stake when one asks if an individual has died is whether or not that individual remains a person in the moral sense, that is, whether or not that individual remains an entity to which we have particular obligations. People in a permanent vegetative state, mentioned above, do not count as dead under the whole brain death definition, but they do count as dead under the higher brain death definition. This dispute about definitions of death, then, has consequences for our obligations (or lack thereof) to individuals in a permanent vegetative state. We will return to this in §3.4.

3.3 THE BADNESS OF DEATH

Many people view death with trepidation. Death, many think, is something we should try to avoid. But why? Is death bad? Medical research and clinical practice are often aimed at prolonging life, or avoiding death. This seems to make sense only if death is an evil to be avoided. Specifying exactly what the nature of that evil is turns out to be tricky. Famously, Socrates held that it is irrational to fear death. Was he right?

Here is a puzzle about the badness of death. Death removes the possibility of all experience, especially of the future, and thus the possibility of any future goods. Whatever it is you care about in life, death entails that you can no longer experience it. This is bad. So in a trivial sense, death is clearly bad. On the other hand, precisely because death removes the possibility of all experience, you cannot, in principle, experience what it is like to be dead. One might think that without the possibility of experiencing a condition, that condition cannot be, for you, good or bad. So death is not good, nor is death bad. So in a trivial sense, death is clearly not bad. (This is an ancient argument, going back to the Roman philosopher Lucretius.) Thus, from the same starting point—that death removes the possibility of all experience—we reach a contradiction regarding whether or not death is bad.

Here's another puzzle about the badness of death, also articulated by Lucretius and discussed in a famous article by Thomas Nagel. Typically, benefits and harms to people occur at particular times. When it comes to the benefits of being alive, this is easy. The particular times that a person benefits from being alive are those times that the person is alive. (At least, the good times! Some would say, the bad times too.) But when it comes to the harms of death, this is not so easy. Death is not symmetric with life on this point: we cannot say that the particular times that a person is harmed from being dead are those times that the person is dead. If that were true, then the harms brought to a person by being dead would, in the long run, approach an infinitely large amount. Supposing that being alive is good, Bach had more of this good than Schubert, because Bach lived longer than Schubert. Supposing that being dead is bad, Shakespeare has received more of this harm than Faulkner, because Shakespeare has been dead for a much longer time than Faulkner. But this is strange. Both of these considerations—that one person can be harmed by death more than another simply because that person has been dead for a longer period of time, and that the harm brought to a person because they are dead approaches infinity as time goes on—suggest that there are no particular moments at which a person is harmed by being dead. Since we tend to think that harms occur at particular moments, one might conclude that death does not harm the person who dies.

Of course, the death of a person can harm others. The death of a spouse, a sibling, a parent, a friend—there is no puzzle that such losses are often tragedies. Such tragedies, though, consist in the harm to *others* when one dies. The above puzzles are about whether or not the person who dies is harmed by their own death.

The badness of death is related to the question about the metaphysics of death discussed in the previous section. There we learned that a person is an individual to whom we ascribe moral status, including various sorts of obligations we have toward that person. It is okay for us to lean against a tree without asking the tree's permission because it is nonsensical to hold that the tree can permit anything, but it is not okay for us to lean against a stranger against their will because the stranger is a person to whom we ascribe a particular status.

A possible solution to the above puzzles about the badness of death is to deny that benefits and harms must come to a person only to the extent that those benefits and harms affect that person directly in space and time. Nagel calls "non-relational" benefits and harms those that directly impact a person as a spatiotemporally bounded individual: eating a delicious meal, conversing with a good friend, and listening to pleasant music are all benefits that accrue to a person at particular moments that require the person to experience those benefits, at those moments, as benefits. Similarly, non-relational harms include getting into a cycling accident, having a nightmare, and listening to a boring lecture: these are events that, if they occur, occur directly to an individual, in that the individual experiences the harm as a harm at a particular place and time.

In contrast, "relational" benefits and harms are those that arise as a relation between a spatiotemporally bounded person and circumstances that do not necessarily coincide with those spatiotemporal boundaries: the keeping of a promise that was made to you even if you never learn about it, the execution of your will after you have died, and the reading of a poem by a stranger to the poet are all relational benefits that accrue to a person but do not require the person to immediately or directly experience those benefits. Similarly, relational harms include being deceived even if one never learns the truth, falling into a coma, or being talked about in hateful terms by others without learning of the conversation.

Consider an analogy. Suppose you state in your will that when you die all of your money should go to a charity devoted to alleviating hunger in sub-Saharan Africa, but after you die your lawyer changes your will such that your money is donated to a local bowling alley. You are not alive to experience this harm, but nevertheless you are harmed. If we agree that there can be relational harms to a person, then perhaps death is such a harm. Death deprives you of the goods of life, even if you cannot experience that deprivation. If we agree that there exist relational benefits and harms (in addition to the existence of non-relational benefits and harms), then death could be such a harm to a person.

Some people find this notion of relational harms to be spooky. Consider the old saying "what you don't know can't hurt you." If there is truth to that saying, it is because perhaps harms are non-relational: they have to happen *to* someone. One might think that a more straightforward way to articulate the badness of death is that one's death guarantees that one's various desires in life cannot be satisfied, and that we ought to prevent and perhaps fear any such event that inhibits the satisfaction of one's desires. This argument, however, is open to the Lucretian challenge: the non-satisfaction of your desires cannot harm you if you are not alive to be harmed.

Let's consider a different thought experiment, made famous by Bernard Williams, which concludes that death is not, in the end, always bad. The thought experiment is based on a play by Karel Čapek, about a woman named Elina Makropulos, whose father had given her a potion to keep her alive forever. She is 342 years old in the setting of the play, and her life has become tedious. Williams suggests that an endless life is a meaningless life. If you were to live long enough, your life would lose the spark and joy and novelty that makes life worth living. Of course, one could radically change one's life projects and develop new fundamental ambitions, in order to fend off boredom. But the more one does this, argues Williams, the more one loses touch with one's identity. One could respond by saying that we can add to our life's ambitions and gradually modify our interests, without necessarily losing touch with our core identity. There is nothing wrong with changing one's identity, and indeed one might think that this can be a very good thing. Indeed, one might argue that the very idea of a core identity is a fiction. But still, there might be a limit to such transformations of our interests and goals. Immortality lasts a long time.

This discussion about the badness of death has been rather abstract. There is, though, a practical and obvious relevance to medicine. Medicine strives to avoid death. A very large proportion of national healthcare budgets is spent on patients who are only days away from death. Some people even have the ambition of immortality. For these projects to make sense, we should have a clear view on whether or not it is a bad thing to die. This question turns out to be harder than many people might think, and we have seen differing answers.

3.4 ETHICS OF KILLING

The title of this section might sound paradoxical or even shocking: how can there be an *ethics* of killing? The belief that killing is clearly unethical is one of the most universally shared moral views. However, most people also believe that killing is not always unethical. Some might think that killing another person in self-defense is permissible, for example, and to take an extreme example, almost nobody thinks that killing an asparagus plant is unethical. Understanding why killing other persons is normally unethical can offer insight into the many difficult sorts of cases that arise in medicine. The ethics of killing in the context of medicine is a core part of medical ethics. The sections on defining death and the badness of death raised several points that are fundamentally related to the ethics of killing in the context of medicine, so we will examine them here.

Consider a patient who has suffered an acute traumatic brain injury and now is in a permanent vegetative state. This diagnosis means that the patient is in an unconscious but partially wakeful state, and after numerous tests and twelve months of monitoring, physicians determine that it is impossible that the patient's cognitive state will improve. Such patients need little life support, because their brainstem is intact, so their cardiac, respiratory, and digestive functioning remain normal, though they need a feeding tube. You might have the intuition that this patient is alive: they are breathing, digesting, and defecating, and they occasionally smile and grunt and shed tears, and their eyes sometimes move around in response to stimuli. However, recall the two different definitions of brain death discussed in §3.2: whole brain death and higher brain death. If you accept the whole brain death definition, then you will consider an individual in a permanent vegetative state to be alive, because their brainstem and other brain functions are intact. If you accept the higher brain death definition, on the other hand, then you will not consider an individual in a permanent vegetative state to be alive, because the patient has permanently lost the capacity for higher brain functioning (especially consciousness). According to the higher brain death definition, an individual in a permanent vegetative state is dead.

Remember that it is not the *organism* that is being assessed as living or dead, but rather it is the *person*. Personhood is the status given to an entity that has particular moral properties, and as noted in §3.2, a strong case can be made that this status should be granted to all and only individuals with particular cognitive capacities, especially the capacity of consciousness. A patient in a permanent vegetative state has forever lost the capacity of consciousness, and thus that person is dead, though the organism remains alive, and importantly, that patient no longer has the moral properties granted to personhood. That patient is due particular forms of respect and care: certainly more care than, say, the desk at which I write this book, and perhaps as much care as, say, one's pet puppy is due, but this patient's status falls short of full moral agency (not primarily because of their diminished physical status but rather because of their diminished moral status).

Keep this patient in mind for a moment, and consider the following. Today there are over 120,000 people waiting for organ transplants in the United States alone, and about thirty people in the United

States die every day because they have not received a donor organ. In the United Kingdom, one person in ten dies while waiting for an organ. A single individual's organs can save the lives of eight people.

These are troubling facts. The defender of the higher brain death definition concludes that patients in a permanent vegetative state ought not be granted moral status. Such individuals are already dead, in the sense that matters (personhood). Thus, concludes this line of reasoning, the organs can be extracted from such individuals and donated to patients on transplant waitlists (of course, usually there are other persons with vested interests that require respect, such as family members, and any such practice would require careful contraints on implementation). This is the case even if the organ extraction brings about the biological death of the individual, because, once again, it is personhood that is the basis of moral status and not the mere fact of being an organism.

Some contributors to the debate about the permissibility or impermissibility of abortion appeal to the same considerations about personhood. Abortion is the cessation of the growth (and, some would say, the life) of a fetus. In a straightforward sense, abortion is the killing of a fetus. Some people take this to be sufficient to conclude that abortion is morally abhorrent. Others, however, argue that killing a fetus does not involve killing a person, because fetuses do not have the necessary attributes of personhood (principally, consciousness). Thus, goes this argument, abortion is permissible. To be clear, not all arguments for the permissibility of abortion are based on the premise that fetuses are not persons, and vice versa, not all arguments for the impermissibility of abortion are based on the premise that fetuses are persons—a famous article by Judith Thompson, for example, grants, for the sake of argument, that fetuses have moral status, and argues that abortion is nevertheless permissible; conversely, an article by Don Marquis argues that although a fetus is not presently a person, it will very likely develop into a person, and so abortion is therefore impermissible. In short, though, a central consideration pertaining to the moral status of abortion is whether or not fetuses are persons.

FURTHER READING

Defining death: McMahan (1995); President's Commission (1981)
Badness of death: Williams (1973), Nagel (1970), Simon (2010)
Ethics of killing: McMahan (2002), Marquis (1989), Thompson
  (1971), Singer (1994)

DISCUSSION QUESTIONS

1. Is an individual who has permanently lost their capacity for consciousness dead?
2. Should medicine strive to keep people alive as long as possible?
3. If an organism dies, does that imply that a person has died? If a person dies, does that imply that an organism has died?
4. Is it okay to extract organs from patients in a permanent vegetative state?
5. Can a person have relational harms or benefits? What does your answer imply about the badness of death?
6. Why are you afraid of death?

PART II

Models and Kinds

4 : CAUSATION AND KINDS

4.1 SUMMARY

In chapter 2 we examined various disease concepts—these are high-level, general theories of disease. Now we turn to models of disease causation and the logic of disease categorization.

To develop a richer understanding of disease causation and categorization it is helpful to know some basics about the general nature of causation. We begin with three fundamental theories of causation, before proceeding to models of disease causation. This discussion of theories of causation is not a complete catalog of theories of causation—that would require its own book—but rather presents a couple of the more intuitive theories that are relevant to the causal models of disease presented later.

Nosology is the study of disease classification. Philosophers have long been concerned with elucidating the basis of "natural kinds." Natural kinds are categories that reflect real divisions in nature. The aim in nosology is to develop disease categories that are natural kinds. One way that medicine strives for this is to base disease categories on the causes of diseases: this is an etiological system of nosology. Another way is to base disease categories on the underlying physiological processes of diseases: this is a pathophysiological system of nosology. Finally, another way is to base disease categories on symptoms of diseases: this is a symptom-based system of nosology.

A key distinction when discussing disease causation is between "monocausal models of disease" and "multifactorial models of disease." Monocausal models of disease identify single necessary and sufficient causes for a particular disease, whereas multifactorial models of disease hold that the causal basis of many diseases is too complex for that. Infectious diseases are often thought of as good examples of monocausal models of disease, while chronic diseases such as type 2 diabetes are often thought of as good examples of multifactorial models of disease. In this chapter we study these two models, and ultimately ask if the distinction is in fact as sharp as it's usually made out to be.

Precision medicine (also called personalized medicine) involves an attempt to define disease categories in the finest-grained way possible, according to knowledge about the etiological and pathophysiological basis of diseases. The basic premise of refining disease categories on the basis of improved biological knowledge is an old one, but today the idea has garnered a great deal of support. We'll examine what exactly precision medicine is, and evaluate its potential for improving medicine.

4.2 THREE THEORIES OF CAUSATION

One view of causation is the sufficiency theory, which holds that a cause is sufficient for its effect (in the right context). For example, if it is raining outside, that is sufficient for me to get wet, and so rain is a cause of my getting wet. Of course, if I have a good umbrella I will not get wet in the rain, which is why we need the context clause added to the sufficiency thesis—rain is sufficient for me to get wet unless I have an umbrella. There are two problems with the sufficiency theory. The first problem is that fully specifying the nature of the context clause, in most real cases, is impossible. I could be wearing a good rain jacket with a hood, in which case I wouldn't get wet in the rain. I could be swimming in a lake, in which case I would already be wet and so the rain would not be the cause of my getting wet. I could be walking in a dense jungle, and so the rain would not reach me through the dense foliage, in which case, again, I wouldn't get wet in the rain. If we cannot specify the nature of the context clause, then the sufficiency thesis will in practice be false. The second problem is related to the first. We appear to have many examples of causes that are in fact not sufficient for their effects, but instead they merely raise the probability of their effects. For example, smoking is not sufficient for lung cancer, but it raises the probability of lung cancer. If you want to hold that smoking is a cause of lung cancer, then, at first glance at least, you have to give up the sufficiency theory of causation.

This latter consideration suggests a second theory of causation: the probability-raising theory of causation. On this account, a cause is anything that raises the probability of something else. For example, unprotected sex with a person with human immunodeficiency virus (HIV) does not guarantee that one will get HIV, but it raises the probability that one will get HIV. The most important nuance that the probability-raising theory of causation must address is the difference between probability-raising features that are mere correlations and probability-raising features that are genuine causes. For example, some studies have found a correlation between eating processed meat and getting cancer. This could be because eating meat in fact raises the probability of cancer, and so on the probability-raising theory of causation, eating processed meat is a cause of cancer. Or, the correlation could be due to a feature of meat eaters such that the link between meat-eating and cancer is noncausal—say, if meat eaters eat fewer vegetables, and the resulting lower dietary intake of fiber was the true cause of cancer.

A third theory of causation, described by J. L. Mackie, has a strange name: the INUS theory of causation. It has this name because a cause, on this account, is an Insufficient but Necessary part of an Unnecessary but Sufficient condition for an effect. Here is a simple example. A match on its own is insufficient to light a fire because you also need fuel (paper, say) and oxygen. A match together with paper and oxygen is sufficient to light a fire. So, a sufficient condition to get fire is the match-paper-oxygen combination: a match is a necessary part of this condition, but alone it is insufficient. The match-paper-oxygen combination is itself unnecessary to make fire, because we could also use a cesium-fluorine combination (please don't try that at home). Thus, a match is an insufficient but necessary part of an unnecessary but sufficient condition for fire. This is an attractive theory of causation, but it faces a similar problem as the sufficiency theory. Consider the smoking-lung cancer example again. What are the other necessary components that smoking has to be combined with such that the combination of smoking and other factors is sufficient to get lung cancer? This is similar to asking what the context clauses are in the sufficiency theory of causation.

The two prominent causal models of disease are the "monocausal model of disease" and the "multifactorial model of disease." With our understanding of general theories of causation, we can investigate these models of disease causation. Although much medical discourse distinguishes diseases as either monocausal or multifactorial, it turns out that it is difficult to ground such a distinction on compelling theories of causation.

4.3 DISEASES: MONOCAUSAL OR MULTIFACTORIAL?

The monocausal model of disease holds that under the right circumstances a particular disease will occur if, and only if, the cause of that disease is present. For example, sickle cell anemia is caused by a single gene mutation at a unique nucleotide. A person who receives copies of this gene mutation from both parents develops sickle cell anemia. All and only people who have two copies of this gene mutation develop sickle cell anemia (though there are other types of sickle cell disease). Or consider tuberculosis: this disease is caused by the bacterium *Mycobacterium tuberculosis*, and all and only people who are infected with this bacterium have tuberculosis.

Diseases of deficiency (such as scurvy, sickle cell anemia, or type 1 diabetes) or diseases of infection (such as tuberculosis or syphilis) are diseases that illustrate the monocausal model of disease. At the end of the nineteenth century and beginning of the twentieth century many diseases like these were discovered, and thus the monocausal model of disease was the paradigm model of disease causation for many years. Famously, the bacteriologist Koch articulated this model of disease in "Koch's postulates," which he intended to be a methodological recipe for discovering the causes of diseases (§9.2).

It can be very powerful to develop monocausal models of diseases because once we know the necessary and sufficient cause of a disease, we can develop interventions to specifically target that cause. For example, once Banting and Best were able to characterize type 1 diabetes as an inability to produce insulin by beta calls in the pancreas, it was obvious that a promising intervention for type 1 diabetes would be to administer exogenous insulin. And indeed, this is one of the most fantastically effective medical interventions, and for this discovery Banting won the Nobel Prize in Medicine (the prize didn't go to Best, because he was just a lowly medical student, though Banting was forced to share the prize with his boss).

The monocausal model of disease is a model of "simple" diseases. However, the issues it raises are far from simple. To illustrate, let's return to the example of tuberculosis. I said that all and only people who are infected with *Mycobacterium tuberculosis* have tuberculosis. This isn't quite right. Only about 10% of people who are infected with this bacterium develop symptoms of tuberculosis. The other 90% have what is called "latent tuberculosis." Indeed, about one-third of the world's population has *Mycobacterium tuberculosis*. If a disease is defined as the total disease entity, including the physiological basis and the symptoms, then people with latent tuberculosis do not in fact have the disease tuberculosis (chapter 2). They simply have one more kind of bacteria in their body, along with the thousands of other kinds of bacteria that do not cause symptoms of disease.

Here the general theories of disease discussed in chapter 2 are relevant. A naturalist should say something like this: it is normal for people to have bacteria in their bodies, and having *Mycobacterium tuberculosis* in one's body is not that rare, and thus latent tuberculosis is not in fact a disease. On this a normativist and hybridist would agree because latent tuberculosis does not cause harm. (Although there is an interesting twist here: latent tuberculosis might not cause physical harm, but it can cause social harm: some people who test positive for latent tuberculosis are denied entry into countries and have their visa privileges revoked.) Because of latent tuberculosis, a monocausal model of tuberculosis is compelling only if we stipulate that infection with *Mycobacterium tuberculosis* is necessary and sufficient for being diagnosed with the disease tuberculosis. But such a stipulation contradicts our general theories of disease. Moreover, it turns out that four other species of *Mycobacterium* can cause symptoms that are virtually indistinguishable from typical tuberculosis. So, it turns out that tuberculosis is not a good illustration of the monocausal model of disease after all, because infection with *Mycobacterium tuberculosis* is neither necessary nor sufficient for developing tuberculosis.

Perhaps a monocausal model of tuberculosis can be salvaged. To deal with the nonnecessity problem, we could stipulate that the various *Mycobacterium* species are causes of different subtypes of tuberculosis: *Mycobacterium tuberculosis* causes tuberculosis$_1$, *Mycobacterium bovis* causes tuberculosis$_2$, *Mycobacterium africanum* causes tuberculosis$_3$, and so on. This partial solution is fine, though it might not be applicable to all kinds of diseases, because for better or worse some diseases are defined symptomatically (as we will see in §12.2, this is especially the case in psychiatry), and for such diseases the subtypes are (presently) indistinguishable based on symptoms alone. We are left with the non-sufficiency problem: infection with *Mycobacterium tuberculosis* is not sufficient to develop tuberculosis because only 10% of people with *Mycobacterium tuberculosis* get tuberculosis. So there is some other factor, call it X, that is necessary, and together with the bacterium, sufficient for causing tuberculosis. In terms of the INUS theory of causation, *Mycobacterium tuberculosis* is an INUS cause of tuberculosis. Why do some people with *Mycobacterium tuberculosis* get tuberculosis and others do not? Because they also have X. Though we do not know what X is, we can postulate its existence to salvage the monocausal model of tuberculosis and carry out research in an attempt to discover what X is.

But if we must stipulate an X factor to explain tuberculosis, does that mean that tuberculosis, in the final analysis, is not a good example of the monocausal model of disease? Wouldn't tuberculosis be better described as a multifactorial disease? That would be hasty. Strictly speaking there are no single causes that are sufficient for their effects. Recall the match-paper-oxygen example from above. A match is not sufficient to start a fire. But a match-paper-oxygen combination is sufficient. All diseases are like this. Consider sickle cell anemia again. In order for the gene mutation to lead to the disease, the embryo with the mutation must develop into a person, the person must not receive a bone marrow transplant, the universe must continue to exist, and so on. In short, there are plenty of necessary conditions—X factors—that must hold in order for the gene mutation to cause the disease. It just so happens that in the case of sickle cell anemia we know what some of those X factors are, whereas in the case of tuberculosis we know less. So, if the presence of X factors entails that a disease is not properly described as a monocausal model of disease—that is, if causes of all diseases are INUS causes—then there are no monocausal diseases, in which case we need a different model of disease.

Alternatively, one could deny the sufficiency aspect of the monocausal model of disease, and posit that there is a fundamental chanciness associated with developing tuberculosis. Of those people who have *Mycobacterium tuberculosis*, 10% get tuberculosis and 90% do not, and that fact, one might say, is simply the result of a stochastic process. On this model of tuberculosis there is not necessarily a hidden X factor, in which case the cause is insufficient for the disease, and thus, again, we need an alternative model of disease.

In the discussion of monocausal models of disease we have already begun to see what a multifactorial model of disease looks like. Many diseases are said to be "complex": a result of multiple causes, such as genes, lifestyle, and environment, working in concert. Cancer, heart disease, and most psychiatric diseases are typical examples. These are sometimes called "chronic" diseases, because they persist for a long duration, as opposed to many infectious diseases, which are aptly described by the monocausal model of disease and which often persist only for days or weeks.

There are a number of possible interpretations of multifactorial models of disease. One is along the lines of the INUS theory of causation. On this interpretation, there are a number of distinct causal factors that all have to be present to bring about a disease. But we have already seen that this is also the case for diseases described by the monocausal model of disease. So if the multifactorial model of disease is based on the INUS theory of causation, there is no real distinction between monocausal diseases and multifactorial diseases.

A related issue is the state of our medical knowledge. One way to understand the multifactorial model of disease is to hold that whether or not a disease is described as multifactorial depends only on our degree of knowledge, or lack thereof, regarding the causal basis of that disease. To call a disease multifactorial or complex is just to say that we do not properly understand the causal basis of the disease.

We could call this the "X factor" interpretation of disease. Like the tuberculosis example in the discussion of the monocausal model of disease, to call a disease multifactorial is just to admit that a given disease has a plurality of causes, some of which we may know and others of which we may not know. These latter causes are the X factors that we have not yet discovered. But just because we do not know what these X factors are does not mean that they do not exist. On this interpretation, so-called complex or multifactorial diseases are ontologically similar to simple diseases such as sickle cell anemia; the difference between multifactorial and monocausal diseases, on this interpretation, is epistemic, in that we know what the X factors are for diseases like sickle cell anemia and we do not presently know what the X factors are for diseases like cancer.

Another interpretation of the multifactorial models of disease is based on a "probability raising" theory of causation. On this interpretation, the various factors identified as causes of diseases are probability raisers of the disease. For example, smoking does not guarantee that one will get lung cancer, but it raises the probability of lung cancer. Such probability raising, on this interpretation, is a brute fact and is not based on our ignorance of X factors. Obviously this interpretation of the multifactorial model of disease does not stipulate that there are no further causes of diseases to be discovered. It simply holds that even if we knew all of the X factors, any single cause in conjunction with its other necessary causes would merely raise the probability of the disease rather than guarantee the disease. But note that this was precisely one of the interpretations of the tuberculosis example, understood as monocausal. So, again, on this understanding there is no sharp distinction between monocausal diseases and multifactorial diseases.

4.4 NOSOLOGY

Nosology is the part of medicine that focuses on how diseases are categorized. We have already seen two kinds of causal models for disease classification: the monocausal model of diseases and the multifactorial model of diseases. The focus of both of these models is on the etiological causal basis of a disease or on the constitutive causal basis of a disease. For instance, infectious diseases can be classified according to the etiological causes of the diseases, namely, the invading bacteria. Other diseases, like type 1 diabetes, are classified according to the pathophysiological or mechanistic basis of the disease (the constitutive causal basis of disease). Still other diseases, like most psychiatric diseases, are classified according to symptoms.

Nosology is about disease categories—how diseases are defined, and what it takes for a person to actually have a particular disease. So it is distinct from diagnosis, which is about inferring what disease a person has on the basis of their symptoms. If one's nosological system is etiological, then there is a sharp distinction between a person presenting with symptoms that are indicative of a disease and that person in fact having that disease. The symptoms are, of course, clues as to whether or not the person has the disease, but symptoms are not conclusive. On the other hand, if one's nosological system is based on symptoms, then there is not much of a distinction between a person presenting with symptoms that are indicative of a disease and that person in fact having that disease. If a disease is *defined* as any case in which a person has symptoms *a*, *b*, and *c*, and then a particular person presents with symptoms *a*, *b*, and *c*, then according to a symptomatic definition, that person has the disease in question.

Most of modern medicine strives toward either an etiological nosology or a mechanistic pathophysiological nosology, or a combination of the two. For instance, type 1 diabetes is a disease in which a person's pancreatic beta cells cannot produce enough insulin, which leads to high blood sugar levels and causes symptoms such as frequent urination, hunger, and weight loss. The inability to produce enough insulin is itself caused by an autoimmune destruction of beta cells in the pancreas, and these beta cells normally produce insulin. Diagnosis, of course, is based on symptoms, such as blood glucose levels after fasting or after a sugar load, and such tests are often performed after other symptoms of diabetes have occurred, such as stroke, slow wound healing, and changes in one's vision. But the disease itself is not defined by such diagnostic criteria. The disease is defined with respect to the mechanistic pathophysiology: type 1 diabetes just *is* the state in which a person's beta cells cannot produce enough insulin.

Many infectious diseases are based on an etiological nosology. For instance, dermatophytosis (ringworm) is a common fungal infection of the skin. Symptoms include athlete's foot, discolored and misshapen fingernails and toenails, and a reddish patch of skin with a slightly darker outside edge. It is caused by about forty types of fungus. For a diagnosis of dermatophytosis, one's skin must be infected by one of these fungi—this is an etiological definition of the disease. So, strictly speaking, dermatophytosis has a many-to-one relation between etiological cause and disease because the disease can be caused by many different species of fungus.

A disease can also be defined with respect to area of the body that is affected. Dermatophytosis is again a good example. Tinea pedis, or athlete's foot, is dermatophytosis of the feet; tinea cruris, or jock itch, is dermatophytosis of the groin; tinea capitis is dermatophytosis of the scalp; tinea barbae is dermatophytosis of facial hair. So in this case etiological nosology is further refined by reference to the particular part of the body that is infected.

Note that dermatophytosis could just as easily be defined by its most salient symptoms, in which case any person who presented with a reddish itchy patch of skin with a slightly darker outside edge, or a discolored and misshapen toenail, would by stipulation have dermatophytosis. Of course, this is how patients are diagnosed, but again, for etiological systems of nosology, a diagnosis is distinct from actually having the disease being diagnosed: diagnosis involves an inference, whereas actually having a disease is a matter of fact independent of one's diagnosis (a physician can be wrong about diagnosing a disease when that disease is defined either pathophysiologically or etiologically). Indeed, symptoms of dermatophytosis can be caused by nonfungal infections, such as bacterial infections, secondary syphilis, pityriasis rosea, or infected eczema. These diseases cannot be treated with antifungal medications, and thus a symptom-based definition of dermatophytosis would be associated with worse treatment outcomes. This is partly why most of medicine aims at either a pathophysiological or an etiological nosology.

However, some domains of medicine employ a symptom-based nosology. Psychiatric nosology is codified in the *Diagnostic and Sta-*

tistical Manual (*DSM*), which is the main handbook of psychiatric diseases, and is now in the fifth edition. There have been historical shifts in psychiatric nosology, from an etiological approach in the early twentieth century, to an "atheoretical" approach with the development of the *DSM-III* in the 1970s, which roughly continues today with the *DSM-5* (the naming of the editions of the *DSM* was based on Roman numerals until the fourth edition; starting with the fifth edition, published in 2013, the *DSM* editions are named using Western arabic numerals). Briefly, the etiological approach to psychiatric nosology involved classifying mental illness according to psychoanalytic theories about the causes of mental illness. But in the mid-twentieth century such theories were no longer thought to be compelling, and so psychiatry moved to what was thought of as an "atheoretical" approach to nosology, which amounted to defining diseases on the basis of symptoms alone. Here is the *DSM-IV* definition of *mental disorder*: "a clinically significant behavioural or psychological syndrome or pattern that occurs in an individual, . . . is associated with present distress . . . or with a significant increased risk of suffering." Think back to our definitions of disease discussed in chapter 2. We see in the *DSM* definition an appeal to symptoms, and specifically to harms of a person with a mental disorder, but not to a naturalistic basis of disease. That is what is meant by the *DSM*'s atheoretical nosology. Moreover, the *DSM* approach to nosology is strictly based on clusters of symptoms and signs (we return to the *DSM* system of nosology in more detail in chapter 12).

Many people find symptom-based nosology problematic. Some psychiatrists and research organizations urge the development of a psychiatric nosology that is etiological or pathophysiological. Even the National Institute of Mental Health has abandoned using the *DSM*. In the place of symptom-based psychiatric nosology, critics urge a pathophysiological basis for psychiatric nosology. In turn, critics of this view hold that a pathophysiological basis for psychiatric theory and practice ignores a great deal of complexity regarding the experience of mental illness—such criticisms are based on a holist rather than reductionist account of disease (I return to this in chapter 6).

A new term for an ancient idea in medicine is called *precision* medicine (sometimes also called *personalized* medicine). Here is how the National Research Council defines it: precision medicine is "the ability to classify individuals into subpopulations that differ in their susceptibility to a particular disease, in the biology and/or prognosis of those diseases they may develop, or in their response to a specific treatment." The basic idea behind precision medicine is to more accurately diagnose patients, using the finest-grained diagnostic categories possible based on microphysiological features of diseases, such as genetic features. The hope is that interventions can target those specific microphysiological features, which would allow therapies to be more precisely targeted—hence the name precision medicine, or medicine being "personalized" to one's specific physiology. So, there is both a diagnostic and a therapeutic aspect to precision medicine. (There is a very different sense of personalized medicine in which the focus of diagnosis and treatment is the person rather than a disease entity—we discuss this in chapter 5.)

The general aim of precision medicine has always been part of medicine. Consider the pathological theory of Galen. Galenic medicine held that our bodies are composed of four fundamental "humors," or elements, and diseases occur when those humors are out of balance. To treat a disease, one first should identify the precise way in which the humors are imbalanced for a particular patient, and then provide treatments that aim to restore humoral balance. As humoral theory was abandoned and new pathophysiological theories took its place, diagnostic specificity and therapeutic precision took on new meanings. In the beginning of the twentieth century the chemist Paul Ehrlich wanted to find what he called *magic bullets* that would specifically target precise disease entities.

Indeed, Ehrlich's goal of finding magic bullets is a good illustration of both the diagnostic and therapeutic aspect of precision medicine. At the turn of the twentieth century there was a coarse-grained disease category called *psychosis*. The term was introduced in 1845 and replaced the older notion of "madness." For a long time one of the most common treatments for madness/psychosis was bloodletting. In 1905 there was an important discovery that allowed one subpopulation of psychotic patients to be distinguished from the rest. The cause of syphilis was identified as the bacterium *Treponema pallidum*. Some syphilitic patients develop "neurosyphilis," which is symptomatically similar to the general state of psychosis. So, from the general population of people with psychosis, medicine was able to identify a subpopulation on the basis of a specific pathophysiological feature, namely, infection with *Treponema pallidum*. Soon after this discovery, Ehrlich developed a chemical that targeted *Treponema pallidum* (this drug was called arsphenamine and was later replaced by penicillin). Thus, the discovery of the constitutive physiological basis of neurosyphilis and its treatment is a paradigm example of precision medicine. (Unfortunately this is one of very few such examples in the history of psychiatry.)

We can understand precision medicine in terms of the monocausal and multifactorial models of disease. Precision medicine aims to improve our understanding of diseases such that those diseases that are now modeled as multifactorial will come to be modeled as monocausal. As noted above, at the end of the nineteenth century and first half of the twentieth century, many diseases that were very important in postindustrial societies could be more-or-less characterized according to the monocausal model of disease. These were infectious diseases like tuberculosis and polio and deficiency diseases like scurvy and type 1 diabetes. Moreover, we were able to intervene on such diseases with great success, using antibiotics, vaccines, improved sanitation and hygiene, and healthier diets. As these diseases became less prevalent (in developed countries at least), other "complex," multifactorial diseases became more important, such as cancer, depression, and heart disease. Our ability to intervene on these latter diseases is poor, at least compared with our ability to intervene on monocausal diseases (see chapter 10). We have good reason to think that we can intervene more effectively on monocausal diseases than we can on multifactorial diseases. Thus, an aim of precision medicine is to learn more about the pathophysiological basis of multifactorial diseases, which will allow us to demarcate subpopulations of current coarse-grained disease categories into finer-grained and ideally monocausal disease categories. In practice, the features that are appealed to today to demarcate subpopulations tend to be based on genetic or other molecular biological properties.

Another way to understand precision medicine is in terms of kinds and categories. To make reliable diagnoses and prognoses, and to intervene effectively on diseases, categories that are constituted by heterogeneous kinds are less reliable than categories that are constituted by homogenous kinds. Consider the example of psychosis again. At the end of the nineteenth century the category "psychosis" included many different kinds of people. On the other hand, the category "neurosyphilis" included precisely one kind, namely, people who had syphilis. At least with respect to the causal basis of the neurological symptoms, this category is composed of a homogenous kind, and this makes the category extremely useful.

Part of the motivation for precision medicine comes from how most medical interventions are evaluated. In chapter 7 we examine the methods for testing medical interventions. The most prominent method is the randomized trial, which involves comparing groups of subjects: a group of patients receives an experimental intervention and a group of patients receives a comparison intervention (either a placebo or a competitor intervention), and then the groups are compared. One worry with such a method is that differences in individuals' responsiveness to treatment get lost in the group analyses. Personalized medicine raises epistemological issues that could influence the way we think interventions should be empirically tested—we look at this in chapter 7.

Another motivation for precision medicine is based on the low effectiveness of many mainstream medications (chapter 10). The hope is that if we are better able to demarcate patient populations according to microphysiological properties associated with their disease, we will be able to develop more effective therapies.

A recent example of precision medicine is the drug trastuzumab (trade name: Herceptin). This drug binds to a receptor called the HER2 receptor. HER2 receptors are signaling proteins in cell membranes that get overexpressed in about a quarter of breast cancers, which leads to excessive cell growth. We can test if a person's breast cancer is overexpressing this receptor, and if and only if it is, trastuzumab can be prescribed as treatment.

The main kind of information used to refine disease categories today is genetic. "Genome-wide association studies" involve comparing the genomes of patients with a disease to the genomes of people without the disease, and looking for differences in the frequency of expression of particular genes. If people with disease d express gene x more often than people without d, then, goes this thought, perhaps x is part of the causal basis of d. The example of neurosyphilis shows that disease categories can be refined by appealing to other kinds of information, but genetic information is the main kind of information now appealed to in personalized medicine. This is probably due in part to the fact that massive amounts of genetic data now can be generated cheaply and quickly.

Some critics argue that there are a number of problems with precision medicine. One is that precision medicine often appears to be committed to a naive form of gene determinism. As just noted, much of the data that is appealed to in order to refine disease categories is genetic. But critics note that there is a very complicated relationship between one's genetic makeup and one's overall physical state. Simply knowing a patient's genetic code is grossly insufficient to be able to precisely prescribe interventions for that patient, at least for the vast majority of diseases. Other critics of precision medicine argue that the treatments that have thus far been developed using this approach are scant and extremely expensive, and in the long run they end up being not much better than already available treatments. For example, the drug ivacaftor is a new treatment for cystic fibrosis, developed with a "precision" approach. Ivacaftor costs hundreds of thousands of dollars per year per patient, and it helps only 5% of patients with cystic fibrosis; whereas low-tech treatments (ibuprofen, aerosolized saline, and an antibiotic) can achieve similar results as ivacaftor and be applied to all patients with cystic fibrosis. Medicine has gone through many trendy movements in its history that promise to revolutionize patient care, and most of the trends fade away. It remains to be seen how helpful precision medicine will be.

Causal models of disease: Carter (2003), Broadbent (2009), Salmon (1997)

Personalized and precision medicine: Green and Vogt (2016), Hey and Kesselheim (2016)

Nosology: Kendler and Parnas (2012), Tsou (2011)

Natural kinds: Khalidi (2013), Lange (2007)

DISCUSSION QUESTIONS

1. Is there a distinction between monocausal diseases and multifactorial diseases?
2. Assess the potential for personalized medicine to modify medical practice.
3. What should be the basis of a disease classification system? Should this apply to all of medicine?
4. What theory of causation best accounts for medical research and practice?

5 : HOLISM AND REDUCTIONISM

5.1 SUMMARY

In the last chapter we saw that much of medicine aims to understand diseases in terms of microphysiological parts and processes. This is *reductionism* about medicine. Medical reductionism holds that diseases should be understood in the finest-grained way possible, by defining diseases according to the abnormal microphysiological parts and processes that constitute diseases, and that medical interventions should target those microphysiological parts and processes. The example of neurosyphilis as an infection by a bacterium and its treatment with a specific chemical is a successful example of reductionism in medicine.

Reductionism in medicine is sometimes called the *biomedical* model of medicine. In the early twentieth century the biomedical model of medicine became widespread, in part thanks to a number of great successes of the biomedical model. Some diseases were aptly characterized by a reductionist approach, and this led to some very effective medical interventions.

Reductionism in medicine ignores the broader contexts in which diseases arise, such as social and economic contexts. Medical reduc tionism has failed to develop effective treatments for a wide range of diseases. Reductionism is associated with viewing patients as mere bodies to be intervened on, rather than people to be cared for. An alternative view is called *holism*. In medicine, holism is a view of diseases, interventions, and patients that attempts to remedy these reductionist shortcomings. Holism considers the object of medical intervention as the whole person rather than a particular disease entity.

Holism has been associated with *vitalism*. Here is a passage from the famous nineteenth-century physiologist Claude Bernard, describing vitalism from the perspective of a reductionist: "Vitalists have always insisted on the impossibility to explain the phenomena of life in physical or mechanical terms; their adversaries have always responded by reducing the manifestations of life to well demonstrated physical-chemical explanations." In contrast to the biomedical model, some people speak of a "biopsychosocial" model, which holds that we must consider more than just the biological features of patients when thinking about and intervening on diseases.

Consider a patient, Sara, who tells her physician that she is suffering after her husband was in a severe car accident two months ago and is now in a coma. Sara has lost interest in her hobbies and is sleeping poorly. She cannot concentrate at her demanding job, which is making her feel guilty and anxious about her next performance review and her ability to pay her husband's medical bills. Sara tells her physician that she is always sad and often finds herself crying. How should we think about what is wrong with Sara? What is Sara suffering from? How should Sara's physician intervene in an attempt to help? Sara appears to satisfy the criteria for being diagnosed with depression (see chapter 12). Does Sara simply have a neuro-chemical imbalance? Should her physician prescribe a pharmaceutical for her? Or, is Sara going through an extended grieving process after her husband's accident, exacerbated by understandable financial and professional stresses? A reductionist views Sara's suffering as a microphysiological problem to be solved by intervening on that microphysiological problem. A holist views some of Sara's suffering as a normal and perhaps healthy part of the human experience. The problem with Sara, says the holist, is more than just a problem with her microphysiological state but is at least as much (or more of) a problem with her whole context, including her husband's accident, her employment, and her healthcare system.

In this chapter we will examine the competing positions of holism and reductionism as they apply to understanding diseases, interventions, and the relationship between physicians and patients.

5.2 DISEASE

In chapter 2 we studied prominent philosophical theories of disease, and in chapter 4 we studied causal models of disease. Here we study two views that differ in their approach to understanding diseases. Reductionists conceive of diseases in terms of microphysiological abnormalities. Holists conceive of disease in broader terms, including the socioeconomic context in which a person suffers and the lived experience of people with diseases (a historical term for holists about disease, particularly in the nineteenth century, was *hygienists* because one of the important factors they considered was hygiene, broadly construed).

There are several distinct disputes between medical reductionists and medical holists. One is ontological: reductionists believe that higher-level properties can and should be reduced to lower-level properties, while holists believe that there are properties at higher levels that cannot be reduced to lower-level properties. An especially illustrative domain for this ontological dispute is psychiatry. Consider depression, for example. Reductionists think that depression is, fundamentally, constituted by microphysiological abnormalities (an old theory, now mostly discarded, was that depression was constituted by a deficiency of monoamines like serotonin). Holists, on the other hand, think that depression cannot be simply reduced to a problem of chemistry. Since there have been virtually no successful reductions of mental properties to physical properties, argues the holist, there is little reason to think that depression can be reduced this way—mental properties like depression are too complex to be reduced and are constituted by, and cause, other higher-level properties that similarly cannot be reduced.

This leads to the second sort of dispute between reductionists and holists, which is methodological. As we will see below, reductionists employ research strategies aimed at discovering the lower-level microphysiological basis of diseases. Conversely, and as would be expected given their ontological dispute, holists think that in many cases this is misguided. Holists believe that we ought to devote more research resources to understanding diseases and interventions at the level at which patients truly experience and suffer from diseases.

There is also an epistemological difference between holists and reductionists that relates to both the ontological and methodological differences. This is about what kinds of explanations are the most apt for particular diseases. Let's continue with the example of depression. Suppose a patient has various symptoms of depression, such as difficulty sleeping, anhedonia, and anxious fidgeting. As we will see in chapter 11, when a physician provides a diagnosis, some people take that to be offering an explanation of a patient's symptoms. So one sort of explanation, which is relatively superficial, is to explain the presence of symptoms by saying that they are caused by the presence of a disease (e.g., "you are having trouble sleeping and suffering from anhedonia because you have depression"). But what explains the presence of depression? Reductionists say that we ought to appeal to lower-level entities and processes to explain the existence of a disease (e.g., "you have depression because you have such-and-such microphysiological abnormality"), whereas holists say that we ought to appeal to the broader context of a patient's life to explain the existence of disease (e.g., "you have depression because your spouse has been in an accident and you have stress at work").

The holist-reductionist distinction about disease only partially tracks the monocausal/multifactorial distinction regarding causal models of disease (chapter 4). Holists think that many diseases are caused by multiple factors, at multiple levels, working together in complex ways, whereas reductionists think that diseases can and should be understood in the simplest terms that the disease in fact allows. But there is nothing in principle about reductionism that commits it to always applying the monocausal model of disease—a good reductionist could discover that in fact multiple causes work together to bring about a disease.

We've seen that psychiatric diseases are an especially acute locus of dispute for holists and reductionists. The psychiatrist Josef Parnas uses the phrase "the ontology of the psychiatric object" to refer to the proper focus of attention for psychiatry. What is the ontology of the psychiatric object? Various answers to this question lie on different parts of the holism-reductionism spectrum. For instance, Parnas himself holds that the ontology of the psychiatric object is the patient's experience. Other psychiatrists, especially those who want a more physicalist basis for psychiatric nosology, hold that the ontology of the psychiatric object is microphysiological entities or processes that constitute diseases (see chapter 12). Some critics of psychiatry hold that the ontology of the psychiatric object shouldn't be the diagnosed person at all but rather should be the (sick) society in which a suffering person lives. At present, diagnostic manuals hold that the ontology of the psychiatric object is the clusters of signs and symptoms that presently define psychiatric diseases. Some holist critics believe that this view of psychiatric diseases ignores a great deal of complexity regarding a patient's experience of her mental illness, including the patient's experience of herself and her relation to her social milieu, the genealogy of her illness, and how her socioeconomic position influences her illness.

For an example of this latter problem, let's again return to depression. In the *DSM-IV*, there was a "bereavement exclusion criterion," which stipulated that if a person was suffering from the recent death of someone close to them, then even if that person was displaying symptoms of depression, that person might not be diagnosed with depression. So in this edition of the *DSM* there was some attempt, however minimal, to take into account one aspect of a person's social context, though note how much of a person's life is neglected: there was no "recently-unemployed exclusion criterion," no "lost-my-life-savings-to-my-gambling-addiction exclusion criterion," no "I-cannot-find-meaning-in-life exclusion criterion," and so on. At the very least the *DSM-IV* took into account this one aspect of a person's context to determine whether a person has depression. But the most recent version of the *DSM*, the *DSM-5*, eliminated the bereavement exclusion criterion. Defenders of eliminating the bereavement exclusion criterion argued that the symptoms of suffering from bereavement are very similar to the symptoms of suffering from depression. Moreover, bereavement can cause depression. Critics of this line of argument make a holist appeal: psychiatry ought to consider a person's broader context when making a diagnosis (we will examine the issue of diagnostic exclusion criteria in psychiatry in more detail in chapter 12). With the above example, such critics argue that a bereaved person who experiences similar symptoms as depressed people very likely does not have the disease of depression but rather is responding normally to a difficult moment in life.

Let's examine the research strategies of holism and reductionism in more detail. This will give us a better understanding of both views and what exactly divides them in their attempt to understand diseases.

The reductionist research strategy aims to understand diseases in terms of the lower-level mechanistic processes that constitute diseases and cause the symptoms of diseases. Medical science decomposes a disease into its component parts and processes, and compares this mechanistic decomposition to the corresponding mechanisms of people without the disease. To understand obesity, for example, the reductionist strives to elucidate the biochemistry of glucose and lipid metabolism in both obese people and healthy people, in an attempt to discover the biochemical basis of obesity.

The holist research strategy, on the other hand, aims to understand disease in broader contexts. Diseases typically do not occur in a vacuum but rather occur in particular social, economic, and lifestyle contexts. Returning to the above example, to understand obesity, the holist strives to understand the social and economic conditions in which people eat unhealthy food and do not get sufficient physical exercise.

In principle these research strategies are not mutually exclusive. Indeed, they are both valuable and arguably are relevant to different sorts of pragmatic concerns. Suppose an alien lands on earth and notices that many people have a rectangular box in their kitchen that they call "toaster." The alien wants to understand toasters. The alien can dismantle the toaster into the smallest pieces possible, keep track of how all the pieces fit together, and develop theories about how the various pieces function. The alien can also observe how people use toasters in day-to-day life. Arguably the alien ought to do both. Suppose the alien begins to use a toaster, and one day it breaks. To fix it, the reductionist strategy would probably be more helpful than the holist strategy. But to understand why it broke in the first place, and how to keep it from breaking again, the holist strategy could be useful.

Both holism about diseases and reductionism about diseases have success stories. Think of the examples that illustrated the monocausal model of disease in chapter 4. Scurvy, syphilis, and tuberculosis can all be well understood in reductionist terms, namely, the etiological or pathophysiological bases of these diseases. These diseases can be diagnosed simply by running a few laboratory tests and then prescribing simple treatments that are highly effective. A reductionist could argue that understanding a person's socioeconomic position or personal situation or experience of their disease adds little to knowing what the disease is and how to cure it. A bacterial infection is a bacterial infection, and one can understand such a disease and successfully intervene on it merely by knowing the microphysiological basis of the disease (in this case, the invading bacteria) and prescribing the right treatment.

On the other hand, holists also have success stories, and some of them involve the very same diseases that the reductionist can cite as a success story. For example, the physician and historian of medicine Thomas McKeown famously argued that tuberculosis rates began to fall long before the introduction of antibiotics and even before we had a reductionist understanding of the causal basis of tuberculosis (namely, the germ theory of disease). The cause of this fall in tuberculosis rates, McKeown argued, was better nutrition, which itself was caused by improved social conditions and better socioeconomic equality. More recently, the epidemiologist Michael Marmot argues that socioeconomic status causes health outcomes: the higher one's socioeconomic status, the better is one's health, and vice versa, the lower one's socioeconomic status, the worse is one's health. Marmot amasses a great amount of evidence to emphasize this holistic aspect of threats to health (we return to the topic of "social epidemiology" in chapter 14).

Reductionism about disease has held sway over medicine since the end of the nineteenth century, after important discoveries like the germ theory of disease. The vast majority of research resources in the medical sciences are devoted to reductionist research programs (chapter 7). In recent years, holism about disease has gained more popularity, thanks to the work of epidemiologists like Marmot.

5.3 MEDICAL INTERVENTIONS

There are competing holist and reductionist views regarding medical interventions. Reductionism about medical interventions focuses on the magic bullet model of interventions, and it is aligned with viewing the targets of interventions as microphysiological entities and processes. Holism about medical interventions argues that other sorts of interventions, such as social or economic interventions, can have great impact on health.

Both holism about medical interventions and reductionism about medical interventions have historical examples of success stories. Thus, like the discussion about holist versus reductionist approaches to disease, one could reasonably say that both holist and reductionist approaches to medical interventions can be important. So, to the extent that there is a dispute, it should be understood not as debating which approach for medical interventions is the right one, but rather, debating where the emphasis for medical interventions ought to be.

Let's start by considering a success story for holism. The argument by Thomas McKeown (mentioned above) is that the decline in mortality in postindustrial nations and concomitant rise in populations was caused less by traditional (reductionist) medical interventions, such as drugs, and caused more by greater socioeconomic equality, which led to improved hygiene and nutrition. This is the influential "McKeown thesis." The successful intervention was holist, in that it involved a complex nexus of social, economic, and lifestyle factors that led to improved health.

More generally, a holist maintains that it is not just the etiological or pathophysiological basis of a disease that should be the target of medical intervention, but also other aspects of a person's life and their surroundings. Consider an obvious example: to increase the mobility of paraplegics and quadriplegics we can restructure their physical environment to maximize wheelchair accessibility, ensuring that sidewalks have curb ramps, buildings have elevators, and public transportation systems have special-use wheelchair vehicles. A reductionist could argue that these interventions are, of course, important, but they are not properly deemed "medical." Medical interventions, on this reductionist line of reasoning, must target the constitutive causal basis of a disease (or disability) or that disease's symptoms. A holist could respond by arguing that this depends on a question-begging distinction between "medical" and "nonmedical" interventions—it's question-begging precisely because holists do not conceive of diseases like reductionists do, as simple physiological abnormalities. Improving wheelchair accessibility increases the health of paraplegics, argues the holist.

Holism can be, then, aligned with a theory of positive health (chapter 1). A neutralist could respond to the above argument by claiming that improving wheelchair accessibility might increase the *well-being* of paraplegics, but this does not increase their *health*, precisely because improving wheelchair accessibility is a modification of the physical context of paraplegics and not their physical state.

Reductionism about medical interventions also has success stories, of course. An example that we saw earlier is a good illustration. The first antibiotic was developed by the chemist Paul Ehrlich at the beginning of the twentieth century, as a treatment for syphilis. Ehrlich coined the term *magic bullet*—he wanted an intervention that specifically targeted a disease entity and eliminated it. The bacterial basis of syphilis had recently been discovered, and Ehrlich's hunch was that a particular chemical could bind to the bacteria and kill it. He eventually found such a chemical, and it proved to be very effective in eliminating the bacterial basis of syphilis and thereby alleviating the symptoms. This is a reductionist medical intervention because it targeted, specifically and potently, the microphysiological basis of the disease.

Ehrlich's magic bullet is just one of many examples of reductionist success stories from that time. A number of important medical interventions were discovered in the first half of the twentieth century, including antibiotics, insulin, and chlorpromazine. In the final decades of the nineteenth century, vaccines were developed for cholera, rabies, tetanus, typhoid fever, and bubonic plague, and now we also have vaccines for polio, measles, diphtheria, and other infectious diseases. Together with theoretical developments, such as the germ theory of disease, the double helix structure of DNA, and highly detailed mechanistic descriptions of normal and pathological physiology, these developments in medicine were all broadly reductionist. Perhaps in part thanks to this recent history of success, reductionism seems to be the dominant approach to medical research and practice today.

Despite these success stories, some people argue that reductionism is now running out of steam. In chapter 10 we study skeptical views of medicine (such as "medical nihilism"), which are in part motivated by a plethora of examples in which reductionism about diseases and interventions seems to be misguided. For example, many diseases that are important today (at least in Western societies), such as obesity or depression, have thus far not been elucidated in reductionist terms, and reductionist interventions for these diseases have been, on the whole, failures. Some people who are critical of reductionism turn to holism and believe that this motivates a different approach to medicine altogether.

Defenders of complementary and alternative medicine often appeal to holism about diseases and interventions to justify their beliefs and practices (see also §10.4). Indeed, a term sometimes used to refer to alternative medicine is *holistic* medicine. Here is a description of holistic medicine from the American Holistic Health Association: "Holistic medicine is the art and science of healing that addresses the whole person—body, mind, and spirit. The practice of holistic medicine integrates conventional and alternative therapies to prevent and treat disease, and most importantly, to promote optimal health." There are several implicit assumptions underlying this appeal to the integration of conventional and alternative medical interventions, and to the importance of positive health (this is suggested by the fact that the promotion of health is stated as distinct from the prevention and treatment of disease).

Stated as a programmatic ambition, holistic medicine aims to accomplish more than merely modulating diseases—it is concerned with the "whole person." But what the whole person comprises according to the above definition appears strange: a person is a body, a mind, and a spirit. Since dualism cannot be taken seriously, let alone "trioism," this appeal to body, mind, and spirit must be understood as a metaphor for various aspects of a person's life, including their values, preferences, and lifestyle (we explore this ambiguous aspect of holism in further detail in the next section). Since standard medicine can, in principle, accommodate people's values, preferences, and lifestyles, then this way of understanding holistic medicine makes it seem very modest.

5.4 PATIENT-PHYSICIAN RELATIONSHIP

The dispute between medical holists and medical reductionists bears on how one ought to think about the relationship between physicians and patients. Should the patient be thought of simply as a semi-reliable reporter of signs and symptoms regarding the microphysiolgical conditions of her body? Or should the patient be thought of, and engaged with, as something more than that?

As we saw above, the dominant approach in medicine is to think of patients as suffering from pathological conditions that are fundamentally reducible to microphysiological abnormalities. Holists claim that this ignores much about the patient's condition. If the patient's condition is just a result of microphysiological abnormalities, then the physician should elicit information from the patient about her symptoms, infer a diagnosis, and prescribe an appropriate treatment that targets the microphysiological abnormality. On the other hand, holists claim that the physician should try to learn much more about the patient's context, should conceive of the patient's condition as more than merely a collection of microphysiological abnormalities, and should prescribe an intervention or set of interventions that addresses the broader understanding of the patient's state.

Holism is aligned with "patient-centered medicine"—this term is meant to highlight a contrast with "disease-centered medicine," which is aligned with reductionism. According to disease-centered medicine, a patient is simply a vessel in which a disease entity exists, and the physician's job is to identify this disease entity and intervene on it, ideally eliminating it. This is a caricature, of course, but it helps to articulate the relevant contrast. Fundamentally, according to disease-centered medicine, the goal of medicine is *to cure*. Patient-centered medicine, instead, is holist: on this view, the whole patient is the focus of medicine, and the physician's job is to engage with the patient as a partner to develop an understanding of the entire life of the patient, including their emotional needs and physical challenges, to focus on overall health promotion and disease prevention, and to foster a mutually respectful relationship with the patient. Fundamentally, according to patient-centered medicine, the goal of medicine is *to care*.

Defenders of patient-centered medicine argue that this approach is more beneficial for patients. Critics of patient-centered medicine argue that this approach needlessly expands the proper domain of medical authority and expertise and is an inefficient use of limited resources (especially the physician's time).

There is an ambiguity about holism noted in the previous section that is pertinent here. Holism might be understood as the requirement that physicians take into account the patient's values and preferences when formulating a treatment plan. Let's call this *values holism*. Or, holism might be understood as the requirement that physicians take into account the broader context of a patient's life when making a diagnosis and formulating a treatment plan. Let's call this *contextual holism*. Or, holism might be a deeper metaphysical view that appeals to the complexity of normal and pathological physiology. Let's call this *metaphysical holism*.

Now let's consider a case. Masha is a competitive badminton player and has a very important tournament in two weeks. Perhaps due to stress from training, pressure from her coaches, or worries about competition, over the last several months she has been having difficulty sleeping, has been irritable and anxious, and has been suffering from headaches and muscle tension. She visits her physician, and the physician diagnoses her with generalized anxiety disorder. They discuss the possibility of Masha taking paroxetine, a selective serotonin reuptake inhibitor (SSRI), to mitigate the symptoms of anxiety. However, the side effects of paroxetine include physical weakness, nausea, diarrhea, and difficulty with sleep. Masha worries that these side effects will impede her performance in the tournament.

According to values holism, the physician ought to take into account Masha's ambitions to perform well at the tournament and thus develop a treatment plan that does not have side effects that could constrain that ambition. Values holism is a modest position, in that it merely requires the physician to consider a patient's preferences and values, and does not commit to particular views about the ontological nature of disease. There is no principled reason a reductionist could not agree with this. According to contextual holism, on the other hand, the physician ought to consider the context in which Masha's symptoms arose, and perhaps suggest that Masha modify this context (for example, perhaps one coach in particular is especially stress-inducing, and she could limit her contact with him). Contextual holism, therefore, expands the domain of medicine relative to reductionism, since a reductionist approach would be to simply diagnose the disease and prescribe the best treatment for it (contextual holism is also more expansive relative to values holism). Finally, it is difficult to say what metaphysical holism stipulates in this case. At the very least, a metaphysical holist should doubt that Masha's anxiety is fundamentally caused by an imbalance in brain chemistry. But what more metaphysical holism demands of the physician is unclear.

There is a final issue about the physician-patient relationship worth mentioning in this context. When you are ill, some of your cognitive capacities can be hindered. Physicians are not just experts, they tend to be healthier than patients, and they have much experience engaging with ill patients. There is a worrying possibility that physicians might view a patient as an epistemic subordinate, in which not only is a patient viewed in the reductionist light as a mere transmitter of information, but moreover, the patient is viewed as an unreliable transmitter of information. This is worrying for both epistemological and ethical reasons: as phenomenologists emphasize, the patient's lived experience is both a crucial source of information and something to be understood in its own right, and engaging with a patient as such is an end in itself.

FURTHER READING

Holism about disease: McKeown (1976), Marmot (2004)
Patient-physician relation: Carel and Kidd (2014), Cassell (1991)
Reductionism: Schaffner (2006), Andersen (2014)

DISCUSSION QUESTIONS

1. Is there a difference in the guidance that holists and reductionists ought to give to physicians when engaging with patients?
2. Is holism about medical intervention a compelling view?
3. Is there a difference in the guidance that holists and reductionists ought to give to medical researchers?

6 : CONTROVERSIAL DISEASES

Is sex addiction a disease? What about "dhat syndrome," a condition found in India in which males worry that they ejaculate prematurely and that they lose semen through their urine? "Hwabyeong" is a condition in Korea characterized by eruptions of anger and symptoms of anxiety and depression, and it is said to be caused by the suppression and buildup of anger in one's body. What about "female sexual arousal disorder," a disease in the *DSM-5* characterizing women who have little interest in sex and receive little pleasure from it? "Running amok" is a type of amnesia in which people go on a killing rampage that they later forget. Or consider a more mundane example, high cholesterol—is that a disease? Indeed, we can ask this about many alleged diseases that our society takes for granted. What about obesity? Social anxiety disorder? Premenstrual dysphoric disorder?

Many diseases in medicine are controversial. Critics claim that some diseases are not "real." This criticism is especially salient in psychiatry. A related claim that some critics make is that normal aspects of human life get "medicalized"—normal human traits get inaptly brought into the scope of medical attention. Another reason some diseases are controversial is the phenomenon of "disease creep," which occurs when standards for diagnosing a disease become easier and easier to meet, rendering more and more people diagnosable with the disease, to the point where healthy people are spuriously diagnosed as diseased.

Some alleged diseases are "culture-bound"—they exist only in a particular time and place—such as dhat syndrome and Hwabyeong noted above. Other examples include "koro" (a condition in Chinese culture in which men have delusions of penis shrinkage as a result of nonsanctioned sexual activity), "couvade syndrome" (a condition originally from medieval Basque culture in which a soon-to-be father experiences symptoms of his wife's pregnancy, including labor pains and even phantom pregnancy-like growth in the belly), and "wendigo psychosis" (a condition in Native American cultures in which a person feels possessed by a spirit and then desires to eat human flesh). These are "culture-bound syndromes."

What does it mean to say that a disease is "real," or conversely, to claim that an alleged disease is not genuine? A disease is a category, or what philosophers call a kind. Some kinds seem to have a natural existence independently of us. Consider the element gold. Anything with an atomic number of 79 is gold, and it will share all the same properties as all other gold: in its pure form it will be slightly yellow, dense, malleable, and it will melt at 1064°Celsius and boil at 2970°Celsius. These properties of gold hold true at all times and places in which the air pressure is one standard atmosphere (ceteris paribus). In other words, the kind "gold" has some essential properties, and those properties are natural.

In contrast, consider the game chess. All games of chess share certain properties: the game is played between two people who start with 16 pieces each, and the game follows certain rules. Like the kind "gold," the kind "chess" has some essential properties, but these properties depend entirely on us. We invented chess. Thus, those properties are not natural.

Finally, consider the category "beautiful music." Obviously the existence of music depends on human activity, so, unlike gold, its properties cannot all be natural. But moreover, there is no essential feature that music must have in order to be beautiful. Some beautiful music is harmonic but not rhythmic, some beautiful music is rhythmic but not harmonic, some has singing, some doesn't. (You might say that one necessary property of beautiful music is that it involves the making of some noise, but you'd be wrong. John Cage, a composer in the twentieth century, wrote the piece titled 4'33", in which the musicians do not play their instruments. He considered it to be his most important composition. Incidentally, this piece sounds a lot like the piece titled "Funeral March for the Obsequies of a Deaf Man," composed by Alphonse Allais in 1897.) Most importantly, because beauty is in the eyes of the beholder, people will disagree about which particular pieces of music ought to be considered "beautiful music."

So, very roughly, the properties that a kind can have can be essential or inessential, and natural or unnatural. When people talk about the reality of a kind, they might have in mind those two features of kinds: whether or not the kind has essential properties, and whether or not the kind is natural. What about diseases? Some diseases seem quite clearly to have essential and natural properties. Consider cataracts, which involve the clouding of your eye lens and are the most common cause of blindness in the world. Cataracts share the property of lens clouding, and exist independently of us and the idiosyncrasies of our categorical systems (even animals get cataracts). So the kind "cataract" is like the kind "gold": it has essential and natural properties.

Alternatively, consider alcoholism. Alcoholics have the property of being addicted to alcohol. But obviously alcoholism could not exist without alcohol, and we manufacture alcohol. So the kind "alcoholic" is like the kind "chess": it has essential but some nonnatural properties (which doesn't fully settle the question of whether or not it is a disease, since as we'll see in §6.5, whether or not addictions are diseases is itself controversial).

Now consider social anxiety disorder. There are a number of symptoms of social anxiety disorder, including fear of being the center of attention, fear of behaving in ways that will be embarrassing, and physiological symptoms that include blushing, sweating, trembling, palpitations, and nausea. But no single one of these symptoms is necessary: a person with social anxiety disorder could have some symptoms but not others, while another person with the disease could have symptoms distinct from the first person. The disease is, arguably, a contingent result of the way our society is structured: zen monks who live alone in caves cannot have social anxiety disorder, and perhaps in societies constituted by happy relationships, free of competition, advertising, stress, and other anxiety-provoking features of society, there would be no social anxiety disorder. Finally, what counts as pathological shyness differs between societies. So the kind "social anxiety disorder" is like the kind "beautiful music": it has no essential properties and it has some nonnatural properties.

Diseases are not just categories. As we learned in chapter 2, diseases are a special set of categories. There are competing theories about what makes disease categories distinct from other categories. These are the theories evaluated in chapter 2: naturalism, normativism, hybridism, and eliminativism. Another angle of critique for controversial diseases is to appeal (implicitly or explicitly) to one's preferred theory of disease. Obviously if there is a dispute about whether or not, say, female sexual dysfunction is a genuine disease, one's view about the dispute should be based in part on a well-grounded general theory of disease and a model of disease causation.

Critics today claim that many alleged diseases are not real diseases. In this chapter we study some of these controversial diseases, and some of the arguments proposed by critics and defenders of these controversial diseases. Some of the more foundational concerns in earlier chapters are pertinent in assessing controversial diseases.

6.2 MEDICALIZATION

People suffer in many ways. Medicine can sometimes alleviate such suffering. When a form of suffering is brought under the gaze of medicine, one might think that this is a positive development. Why not help people however we can, including with the use of tools that medicine has at its disposal?

Sometimes scientists, companies, and patient advocacy groups urge medical organizations and regulators to take more seriously a condition that is not yet recognized as a legitimate disease. Critics claim, however, that very often the "medicalization" of otherwise normal aspects of life, even painful aspects that involve suffering, is unwarranted and can lead to nefarious consequences. Here is a passage from an article in the *British Medical Journal*, warning against the risks of medicalization:

> Inappropriate medicalisation carries the dangers of unnecessary labelling, poor treatment decisions, iatrogenic illness, and economic waste, as well as the opportunity costs that result when resources are diverted away from treating or preventing more serious disease. At a deeper level it may help to feed unhealthy obsessions with health, obscure or mystify sociological or political explanations for health problems, and focus undue attention on pharmacological, individualized, or privatized solutions. (Moynihan, Heath, and Henry 2002)

There are many examples of alleged diseases that critics claim have been inappropriately medicalized. Present-day examples include attention deficit hyperactivity disorder, female sexual dysfunction, most cases of depression, obesity, and addiction. History provides more examples. In the nineteenth century there was a disease called "drapetomania," which was defined as slaves having the symptom of wanting to escape from their masters—in this case an important political issue was medicalized. Masturbation used to be considered a disease, as did homosexuality. Some critics of medicalization claim that medicalization involves an attempt to control deviant behavior—behavior that is not consistent with social, religious, patriarchal, or capitalist norms—rather than an attempt to alleviate the suffering of people with genuine diseases. We return to this in chapter 12.

Critics of medicalization note that too often the underlying motive for medicalization is the financial profit of companies that manufacture interventions for the condition being medicalized or the financial profit of professionals responsible for treating the condition. The derogatory term for the medicalization of a condition for financial gain is "disease mongering." There are prominent recent examples of medicalization being motivated by corporations. Consider "female sexual arousal disorder" (or "female sexual dysfunction"). As noted above, this condition affects females who experience an ongoing lack of interest in, and absence of pleasure from, sex. Because of the great success of the drug Viagra, which helps mitigate erectile dysfunction in men, companies have been looking for a "female Viagra"—a pill to sell to females to enhance their sexual life. But in order to market a new drug for a condition, that condition must first be recognized as a disease. So companies became involved in a number of activities aimed at getting "female sexual dysfunction" recognized as a disease, which they succeeded at. Recently a pharmaceutical, flibanserin, was introduced that has a small effect on symptoms of female sexual dysfunction, and the manufacturer of the drug funded patient advocacy groups to demand that the US Food and Drug Administration (FDA) approve the drug.

One could respond to this critical position by noting that some women do in fact have little interest in sex, and since sex is an important aspect of life, such women experience a significant harm from their condition. At least according to a normativist theory of disease, such women might have genuine diseases. If so, then there is nothing intrinsically pernicious if physicians, regulators, and corporations codify the condition and attempt to develop interventions for it. Indeed, one might say that this is a benevolent act.

On the other hand, according to a naturalist or hybridist theory of disease, there must be a pathophysiological basis to female sexual dysfunction if we are to consider it a genuine disease. Even if it is a genuine disease, there is a separate question about what the best way to treat the disease is. Sometimes critics of medicalization take a holist stance against what they take to be an excessively reductionist position about significant aspects of the human condition (chapter 5). On this view, female sexual dysfunction might be a genuine disease, but to conceive of the disease in pathophysiological terms ignores the crucially important social context of female sexuality, and treating the disease with a reductionist intervention (a pharmaceutical) is less effective than treatments that take into account the whole social and personal context of women. There is now a reductionist intervention for male sexual function that is arguably very effective (though whether or not this intervention is used for genuine diseases in most cases is another question), but that does not entail that a reductionist approach to female sexual function will be effective. Some aspects of female sexuality may be more complicated than male sexuality and require a "holist" approach to understand it and effectively intervene.

A phenomenon related to medicalization is "disease creep," which occurs when the diagnostic criteria for a disease, or a pre-disease state, are weakened, thereby becoming easier to satisfy, which entails that more people become diagnosable with the disease. Many diseases and pre-disease states are diagnosed by measuring physiological parameters such as blood pressure or cholesterol levels. One way in which disease creep occurs is when the diagnostic thresholds of these parameters are lowered. Hypertension is a good example. Hypertension is a long-term state of high blood pressure, which is a risk factor for strokes and heart attacks. The blood pressure level for what counts as hypertension has tended to be lowered over time, which renders more people categorized as having high blood pressure.

Disease creep is exacerbated by the practice of diagnosing "pre-disease" states. Hypertension again provides a good example. Physicians now diagnose a condition called "pre-hypertension," which amounts to having a close-to-normal blood pressure, albeit slightly on the high side. Defenders of lowered diagnostic thresholds argue that such lowered thresholds are precautionary—diagnosing a person with pre-hypertension earlier rather than later can help them avoid full-blown hypertension and possibly a heart attack. Critics of "disease creep" argue that lowered diagnostic thresholds merely benefit pharmaceutical companies—if more people are diagnosed with hypertension, then more people will consume drugs to lower their blood pressure. These critics argue that the empirical evidence suggests that such drugs do not help people diagnosed with the lower thresholds, and they point to conflicts of interest in the committees that formulate the thresholds (in the case of hypertension, many of the committee members have had financial ties to companies that manufacture drugs to lower blood pressure).

There is another angle of medicalization to consider. Recall that critics of medicalization claim that too many cases of various forms of human suffering come under the gaze and control of medicine. To take another example, a prominent book is titled "The Loss of Sadness"—the authors argue that too many cases of normal human sadness have been inappropriately medicalized as depression. However, many people claim that diseases should be "normalized" so that people who suffer will not feel stigmatized by their condition and will be more willing to disclose their suffering to others and to seek help. This concern is especially pressing for diseases that are stigmatizing, such as psychiatric diseases and various disabilities. Depression is again a good example: some people suffer from depression quietly, without admitting to themselves or other that they are suffering, but if they were less afraid of being stigmatized they might be more willing to seek help. To respond to such stigmatization, patient advocacy groups and others promote the "awareness" or normalization of certain diseases. Of course, awareness-raising normalization of a disease can contribute to the medicalization of the disease. So if one is opposed to such medicalization, one may inadvertently be opposed to the aim of de-stigmatizing forms of suffering. Thus there is a tension between the two aims of wanting to avoid the inappropriate medicalization of conditions and wanting to avoid the stigmatization of harmful conditions.

6.3 PSYCHIATRIC DISEASES

Controversy about psychiatric disease categories is widespread, and we have already mentioned several examples in previous sections and chapters. Do fidgety young boys have a disease called "attention deficit hyperactivity disorder"? Should a person who is grieving after the death of her spouse and who has many of the symptoms of depression be diagnosed with depression, or be excluded from this diagnosis on the grounds that she is grieving? Are psychiatric disease categories coextensive with specific abnormalities of brain physiology, or is the relation between the constitutive causal basis of psychiatric diseases and the way these diseases are classified based on symptoms more complex?

Controversy about psychiatric diseases is sometimes based on differing views about nosology, which we studied in chapter 4. Controversy about psychiatric diseases can arise from particular alleged disease categories, like those noted above. As we saw in the previous section, some critics claim that most cases of depression are normal (and not diseased) responses to life's difficulties. Controversy about psychiatric diseases can arise because of the phenomenon of medicalization, discussed earlier. For example, consider the alleged disease premenstrual dysphoric disorder, which was added to the *DSM-5* in 2013. This is an especially harmful version of premenstrual syndrome—symptoms include irritability, depression, mood lability, anxiety, and fatigue, and physical symptoms like abdominal bloating, breast tenderness, and headaches—but some critics claim that such symptoms are typical features of menstruation. Controversy about psychiatric diseases can arise from disputes about the general nature of disease. Consider the claim that critics make about premenstrual dysphoric disorder: if one is a normativist about disease, all that matters in holding that premenstrual dysphoric disorder is a genuine disease is that it causes some women to suffer. That alone warrants calling it a genuine disease, says the normativist. (How would a naturalist respond to this?)

Many psychiatrists themselves debate particular disease categories and the general quality of psychiatric nosology. For example, the psychiatrist Kenneth Kendler argues that although psychiatry is in its infancy and its categories are only "first approximations," psychiatry has made plenty of progress, and he invokes what philosophers call the *no miracles argument* to argue that such progress would not have been possible if psychiatric classification was fundamentally flawed. Critics, however, deny that psychiatry has made much progress, and so for such critics this argument is not very compelling. A long history of nosological and therapeutic failures in psychiatry ought to make us doubtful of present psychiatric categories and treatments, goes this critical line of reasoning. We will return to this in chapter 12.

There is an additional feature about psychiatric categories, articulated by Ian Hacking, that is cause for concern. Psychiatric categories are "human kinds"—categories that are studied by the human sciences, such as psychology, sociology, anthropology, and psychiatry. Suicidal people, homosexuals, addicts, and university professors are all examples of human kinds. Hacking argues that human kinds have "looping effects": people who are classified as a member of a human kind change as a result of their classification. This change may be due in part to their own conscious awareness that they have been classified, and it may be due in part to other people treating them differently as a result of their classification. The net effect is that individual members of a human kind change in virtue of their classification as members of this kind. This in turn entails that the human kind itself changes (because token elements of the kind have changed). And this in turn entails a couple of worrying phenomena: some features of that kind may become artificially solidified, and knowledge of that kind developed by the relevant human science will be unstable. Spiders, gold, and distant stars, in contrast, lack such a looping effect. To put the idea in terms from above, Hacking concludes that human kinds are different from natural kinds, and this is important because natural kinds feature in natural laws and support inductions, predictions, and explanations. If Hacking is correct that the looping effect of human kinds entails that human kinds are not natural kinds, then human kinds cannot serve the same role as natural kinds in these important epistemic activities.

Some critics of Hacking's argument have doubted that there is a sharp difference between human kinds and natural kinds in the way that Hacking claims. The properties of some natural kinds also change as a result of their classification. For example, because marijuana has been classified as an illegal plant, the plant is now often grown indoors using artificial lighting, and token members of the kind have changed as a result—this natural kind has a looping effect. Of course, Hacking could reply that plants do not become aware of their classification in the same way that, say, addicts do. This response raises the further question of how exactly looping works—in what sense does the feedback from being classified have to affect token members of a kind such that human kinds (like the category "addict," say) are not natural kinds (like the category "marijuana plants," say)? This is one of many questions about Hacking's interesting argument about the looping effect of human kinds—it has generated a lot of commentary among philosophers.

6.4 CULTURE-BOUND SYNDROMES

Some diseases seem to occur only in very particular contexts. For example, one of the first cases of multiple personality disorder was in the 1960s, and in the 1980s many thousands of cases of multiple personality disorder were diagnosed in the United States, but then the frequency of cases dropped off, and now the *DSM* does not even list multiple personality disorder as a disease. A more recent example is *uppgivenhetssyndrom*, or refugee resignation syndrome, which exists only in Sweden and only among refugees and only among children and adolescents and only in the past two decades; symptoms include withdrawal from daily life as well as a lack of eating and talking and hygiene, and the cause typically involves trouble with the refugee family maintaining legal residency status in Sweden. The examples that I started this chapter with—dhat syndrome, hwabyeong, female sexual arousal disorder, and running amok—are culture-bound syndromes. There are many of these alleged diseases throughout the world.

Such diseases are controversial. The Swedish refugee resignation syndrome is a good example. Critics of the practice of diagnosing refugee children with the syndrome claim that the children are faking the symptoms in order to help their families attain legal residency in Sweden. Defenders of the practice retort that such critics are xenophobic and racist.

The admission that culture can be responsible for the existence of a disease or at least important features of a disease is troubling for the view that diseases are simply objective and natural features of the world. The very fact that such states are "culture-bound"—that is, confined to very local cultures—might suggest that such states are not genuine diseases. Moreover, it makes one wonder: are any of our own culture's diseases culture-bound? Mainstream (Western) psychiatry claims that the answer to this question is "no": the assumption is that diseases as defined by the *DSM* are universal. Of course, the *DSM* is not an infallible nosological guide, as suggested by the previous section and chapter 12. And Western psychiatry has had its fair share of alleged diseases that were temporally transient, such as multiple personality disorder, or that were considered to be a disease at one time and then later not, such as homosexuality. In any case, culture-bound syndromes are discussed in the *DSM*. In the *DSM-IV* the definition of a *culture-bound syndrome* was "recurrent, locality-specific patterns of aberrant behavior and troubling experience that may or may not be linked to a particular *DSM-IV* diagnostic category."

Some culture-bound syndromes are quite strange. Ode-ori, in Nigeria, is a feeling that one has parasites crawling inside one's head, and it is accompanied by a fear of being attacked by evil spirits. Hwabyeong, "anger illness" or "depression anger illness" in Korea, is a frustration from a perception of unfairness, and comes along with physiological symptoms such as fatigue, abdominal pain, palpitations, insomnia, and anorexia. Hwabyeong sounds a lot like what Western psychiatry would call anxiety or depression. Of course, it is possible that our anxiety and depression are just as bound to our culture as hwabyeong is bound to Korean culture. This is not to say that such diseases (those of other cultures or of ours) are not real, but just that their existence or at least details of their presentation are determined by contingent facts about particular cultures.

Why are culture-bound syndromes "bounded"? Their bounded-ness, along with their strangeness, calls out for explanation. That is, why do some of these alleged diseases occur in very particular socio-cultural circumstances?

A skeptic about culture-bound syndromes has a ready explanation: culture-bound syndromes are bounded because they are not real, genuine diseases. Genuine diseases do not respect national bound-aries or exist in very particular temporal periods; unlike culture-bound syndromes, bacterial infections, type 1 diabetes, and cancer are going to be around as long as humans are around, wherever humans happen to be (unless, as seems very unlikely, medicine can finally eliminate these diseases altogether).

This skeptical explanation is tempting but should be resisted. Al-though some paradigmatic examples of disease, such as those men-tioned just now, are relatively unbounded in space and time, it is an excessively strong requirement that particular diseases must be spatio-temporally unbounded. In a trivial sense, all human diseases are spa-tiotemporally bounded, merely in virtue of the fact that human exis-tence is spatiotemporally bounded, and human existence is a necessary condition for human diseases. Skeptics of culture-bound syndromes could readily accept this and nevertheless respond by stipulating that the spatiotemporal boundary of a genuine disease ought to coincide with the spatiotemporal boundary of human existence. But even this is an excessively strong requirement. Think of diseases that have arisen naturally at some point in human history (for example, AIDS), or dis-eases that have arisen as a result of technological developments (such as addictions or gunshot wounds), or diseases that have been eradi-cated (at the time that I am writing this, smallpox is the only example of a human disease having been eradicated, but experts predict that other infectious diseases will soon be eradicated).

Perhaps what the skeptic ought to say is that genuine diseases are relatively unbounded in space and time, whereas culture-bound syndromes are very spatiotemporally bounded. But how unbounded does a disease have to be for it to be real, according to the skeptic? Suppose an extremely rare genetic mutation arises in just one person in all of human history, and this mutation causes extremely harmful symptoms—it satisfies any of the definitions of disease discussed in chapter 2, yet only affects a single person during a relatively thin slice of human history, and so is extremely bounded.

There is another reason to resist straightforward skepticism about culture-bound syndromes, suggested in this example of a rare genetic mutation that causes great harm. All culture-bound syndromes cause harm. So at least according to normativism about disease, culture-bound syndromes are, *by definition*, real diseases. This is not a decisive argument, of course, because you might not agree with normativism about disease—you might be a naturalist or hybridist, in which case you would require a culture-bound syndrome to have a biologically abnormal underpinning in order for it to be a genuine disease.

Straightforward acceptance of culture-bound syndromes as genuine diseases—call this *realism* about culture-bound syndromes—also seems misguided. There really does seem to be a difference in kind between conditions like type 1 diabetes and conditions like dhat syndrome. Perhaps the difference can be articulated by noting the problems that critics have raised for normativism about disease. One criticism is that normativism is too expansive regarding the proper domain of medical expertise and authority. "Running amok" sounds like a strange disease to our ears precisely because killing rampages are not in the proper domain of medical expertise. Another criticism was noted a moment ago: normativism does not require a biological basis of disease. Ode-ori sounds like a strange disease to our ears because we have no idea what the biological basis could be for the feeling that one has parasites crawling inside one's head. These challenges to realism about culture-bound syndromes are also indecisive. For all we know, ode-ori could be rooted in a biological abnormality, and it's just a historical contingency (though a rather reasonable one) that killing rampages are not managed by physicians.

Ian Hacking has been among the most prominent commentators on culture-bound syndromes. Examples that he has written extensively on include fugue (a condition that affected young men in nineteenth-century France and that involved wandering aimlessly from town to town), multiple personality disorder, and *uppgivenhetssyndrom*, the refugee resignation syndrome. Hacking has suggested an explanation of culture-bound syndromes that attempts to forge a compromise between skepticism and realism. His explanation depends on a notion introduced in the previous section: looping effects. The idea is that culture-bound syndromes begin with a few initial real cases that involve genuinely strange and harmful conditions. Because of their novelty and severity, these cases get plenty of attention from the medical community, media, friends, and family.

Here's the idea. An initial category (such as "refugee resignation syndrome") is formulated by experts. The category becomes a condition. People learn of this condition and come to understand, implicitly or explicitly, that this condition is a way humans can be. You could have this condition, or your child could have this condition, or a patient under your care could have this condition. You start to look for symptoms, in yourself, in your family members, in your patients. Some people begin, unconsciously, to fashion themselves after this condition. This is a form of mimicry, but it is not necessarily mischievous or deceptive—it is more like the mimicry of style (as when many university professors over the age of fifty seem to dress similarly). More cases develop, and so the condition gets more attention. The condition becomes an epidemic. At some point, usually within a generation or so, the number of new cases dwindles, and for some culture-bound syndromes the condition altogether disappears.

There is something compelling about Hacking's explanation of culture-bound syndromes. However, it leaves some perplexing questions unanswered. For example, refugee resignation syndrome occurred only in Sweden, only among refugee children from very particular regions, and almost exclusively among the first-born child in a family; the symptoms were severe, involving a near-comatose state for months; the most effective intervention for the condition was the granting of legal residency status to the family of the child suffering from the condition. These are strange facts. Consider the specificity of both the region where the condition occurred and the regions from where the refugees originated. There is little about Hacking's model that explains such specificity.

6.5 ADDICTION

There are two dominant theories about addiction. One theory claims that addiction is a disease: addiction is constituted by chemical changes to normal brain physiology, leading to dependence on exogenous substances brought about by repeated consumption of those substances—this is the *disease* theory of addiction. The disease theory of addiction is sometimes referred to as the "biomedical model" of addiction. This theory emphasizes the poor self-control that addicts display and the physiological aspects of substance dependency. Another theory claims that addiction is not a disease, but rather is a set of harmful behaviors brought about by a series of bad choices—this is the *moral* theory of addiction. This theory emphasizes the fact that addiction in a literal sense is constituted by a series of choices, and that addicts in principle have agency and they exercise that agency poorly.

One argument for the disease theory of addiction is that repeated use of a particular substance that leads to dependence comes along with associated neurophysiological changes. It is a paradigm case of a condition that has an exogenous physical cause (overuse of substances) and a biological constitutive basis (the associated brain changes). Specifically, addiction involves changes to the mesolithic dopamine system. So addiction is like type 1 diabetes or bacterial infections in that there is a microphysiological basis of the condition. This suggests that addiction is a disease. A response to this argument is that similar brain changes can be brought about by learning a musical instrument or developing a physical hobby such as rock-climbing. Since it is unintuitive to think that these activities are diseases, it follows that mere brain changes associated with a behavior are insufficient for that behavior to be deemed a disease. Thus the brain-change argument for the disease theory of addiction is not compelling.

There is a similar argument for the disease theory of addiction that notes that there is empirical evidence that suggests that addiction has a genetic basis. Proclivity to addiction is, in part, heritable. So, in this sense, addiction is like sickle cell anemia, cystic fibrosis, muscular dystrophy, Alzheimer disease, phenylketonuria, and many other uncontroversial diseases. This suggests that, at least according to naturalism about disease, addiction is a disease. Since addiction is so obviously harmful to addicts, normativism and hybridism about disease concurs with naturalism. However, quite obviously a great many of our physical and behavioral features have a genetic basis, and yet these features are not diseases—think of eye color or athletic prowess.

Still another argument for the disease theory of addiction is based on the phenomenology of addiction. Once one becomes addicted to a drug, the desire for that drug is extremely intense. This desire is typically irrational, and not just from a third person observer but also from the first person perspective of the addict herself. Many addicts want the drug that they are addicted to so much that they are willing to sacrifice their friendships, family relations, and careers to get access to the drug. Addicts can be aware of these great costs, and can know that withdrawal is difficult but not always that bad, and can know the drug does not bring them much pleasure, and still, despite all this knowledge, their desire for the drug is strong. This suggests that addicts have lost self-control, that the possibility of real choice for addicts is extremely limited, and that their state is truly pathological. This appeal to the phenomenology of addiction is indecisive, since similar patterns of behavior can arise in other domains of life. Think of a tennis star like Andre Agassi, who made immense personal sacrifices to become a great tennis player, despite the fact that he did not really enjoy playing tennis very much, and though it often caused him profound anguish, he kept doing it.

The moral theory of addiction holds that addiction is a moral failing—it arises from a series of poor choices, which are made as a result of abnormal desires, mistaken beliefs, or both. Addiction begins, in a superficial sense, by an individual making a series of choices. To become an addict one must make choices, goes this thought—to drink alcohol or smoke cigarettes or snort cocaine—not once or twice but many times over an extended period. Since personal choice is so central to addiction, this suggests that addiction is not a disease but is rather a prudential failure. In contrast, one does not choose to get type 1 diabetes, cancer, or infection. This line of reasoning is not much of a consideration in favor of the moral theory of addiction because many diseases begin as a result of a person's choices. Food poisoning is a result of a person choosing to eat bad food, an injury suffered from skiing is a result of a person choosing to ski, and obesity is often the result of poor dietary choices. Even phenylketonuria, a condition caused by a simple genetic abnormality, cannot cause symptoms unless a person chooses to consume food with phenylalanine in it. Thus, the argument for the moral theory based on the fact that the genesis of addiction involves an individual's choices is not compelling.

Another problem with this argument for the moral theory of addiction is that it is committed to the view that humans have the capacity to make genuinely free choices—that humans have free will. Of course, many people believe deeply that we do in fact have free will. But this is controversial. The choice to open a beer might not be, in a fundamental sense, a choice at all, but rather might be the result of a complex set of neurophysiological events. If all apparent choices—including both benign quotidian choices like brushing your teeth, to imprudent addiction-generating choices like snorting cocaine—are at bottom just a result of your neurophysiological activity, then it seems strange to say that addiction is the result of poor choices. Rather, addiction is the result of neurophysiological activity (goes this argument), just like brushing your teeth and solving logic puzzles. This is hardly a decisive consideration against the moral theory of addiction, since whether or not humans have free will is, to say the least, an unsettled debate. But the commitment to free will is some intellectual baggage that the moral theory must carry.

A less abstract and philosophically controversial version of this concern about free will is based on the phenomenology of addiction. The act of consuming the drug that an addict is addicted to is often not motivated by deliberation. The link between addictive desire and consumption is often not mediated by much thought at all—rather, the link between desire and action for addicts is in many cases direct. An alcoholic simply pours himself another drink. This is very different from, say, choosing what to have for dinner, which book to read, or where to go on holiday.

A better argument in favor of the moral theory of addiction is that addicts respond to incentives. For example, certain professional groups, such as airline pilots, have strong incentives to avoid addiction. If a pilot is identified as being addicted to a drug (including alcohol, of course), she is required to cease consumption of that drug and to take regular drug tests. If she were to fail these tests she would be fired. The financial stakes of this are high. Such pilots are good at ceasing to consume whatever substance they were addicted to. Other addicts appear to respond to more modest positive incentives. For example, many cocaine addicts stop using cocaine when they are offered small cash rewards if they provide clean urine samples on a regular basis. In short, much evidence suggests that even addicts are able to display some self-control. If addicts choose not to consume the substance that they are addicted to when they are offered incentives not to, this suggests that when addicts do consume the substance they are addicted to it is a choice made just like most other choices, involving an implicit weighing of costs and benefits, rather than a compulsive action lacking self-control. Insofar as it is a choice, it can, like all other choices, be judged. At the very least, goes this thinking, addiction-conducive choices are imprudent. At the very worst, addiction-conducive choices are immoral: they sap a person's dignity and freedom, harm others for selfish gain, and are extremely wasteful.

The moral theory of addiction cannot be the view that the addictions of *all* addicts are a result of poor choices. There are cases of people being forced to consume addictive drugs against their will. These people then develop a chemical dependency. To hold such people responsible for the genesis of their addiction is entirely implausible; to hold such people responsible for the ongoing use of the drug is not as implausible, but nevertheless seems naively unsympathetic to the power of chemical dependency.

Perhaps in part because addiction can appear to be a moral failing, one dominant tradition of treating addiction has been, broadly construed, moral. Alcoholics Anonymous has been the dominant approach to treating addiction for close to a century. Alcoholics Anonymous bases its approach on religious principles, encouraging their members to devote themselves to a "higher power" to help alleviate their "defects of character." The "bible" of Alcoholics Anonymous claims: "Rarely have we seen a person fail who has thoroughly followed our path. Those who do not recover are people who cannot or will not completely give themselves to this simple program, usually men and women who are constitutionally incapable of being honest with themselves." (There is now a vigorous debate about the effectiveness of Alcoholics Anonymous, based on many of the epistemological issues that we will study in chapters 7 and 9, though certainly many people claim to have controlled their addictive behavior thanks to this program).

Addiction is, of course, stigmatized by society. It is without a doubt a terrible condition for a person—addiction causes great harm to addicts. But this is not much of a consideration for the moral theory of disease, since many diseases are also stigmatized, such as sexually transmitted diseases, obesity, and leprosy. Moreover, according to normativism and hybridism about disease, a condition *must* cause a person harm, so the fact that addiction is harmful to an addict is not a consideration in favor of the moral theory of addiction but is rather a consideration in favor of the disease theory of addiction, from the perspectives of normativism or hybridism about disease.

Some theorists attempt to articulate a middle theory that accommodates the range of considerations above. There is a trivial sense in which a condition can be both a moral failing and a disease. For example, if I get drunk and then go skiing and get into an accident that breaks my leg, my condition is the result of an imprudent choice and yet is obviously a condition that is the proper target of medical care (injuries are diseases in the broad technical sense of the term used in philosophical discussions). I leave it to you to determine whether a theory of addiction can be developed that renders the considerations that motivate the disease theory of addiction consistent with the considerations that motivate the moral theory of addiction.

FURTHER READING

Medicalization: Illich (1975), Horwitz and Wakefield (2007)
Culture-bound syndromes: Hacking (2010)

Addiction: Pickard (2015), Holton and Berridge (2013)

Looping effect of human kinds: Hacking (1995), Cooper (2004), Tsou (2007), Kuorikoski and Pöyhönen (2012), Tekin (2014)

DISCUSSION QUESTIONS

1. Choose your favorite controversial disease. Is it a genuine disease? Explain.
2. Are diseases relative to particular cultures, or are diseases "universal"?
3. Is addiction a result of weakness of will, or is it a disease?
4. Are the kinds studied by the "human sciences" fundamentally different from the kinds studied by the "natural sciences"?

PART III

Evidence and Inference

7 : EVIDENCE IN MEDICINE

7.1 SUMMARY

Biomedical science studies many different sorts of questions, including the physiological basis of diseases, the causes of diseases, and the frequency of diseases in various populations. One of the most important types of research in medicine is to find effective ways to intervene on diseases. In this chapter we investigate philosophical problems that arise in the context of research that is directed toward assessing the effectiveness of medical interventions.

For typical hypotheses regarding the effectiveness of pharmaceuticals there is evidence from computational models, studies on cells and tissues, experiments on multiple animal species, multiple kinds of epidemiological studies of human populations, randomized trials, and summaries of the primary evidence by meta-analysis. The evidence-based medicine (EBM) movement assesses this diversity of evidence with evidence hierarchies, which are rank orderings of kinds of research methods according to the potential for those methods to suffer from bias. This ordering is usually determined by one or very few parameters of study designs. Systematic reviews and meta-analyses are typically held to be at the top of such hierarchies, randomized controlled trials (RCTs) are near the top, non-randomized cohort and case-control studies are held to be lower, and near the bottom are laboratory studies and anecdotal case reports. Studies on animals play an important role in branches of medicine such as toxicology, but the extent to which we can extrapolate from findings in animals to conclusions in humans is controversial.

In short, there is a great diversity of evidence available to assess the effectiveness of medical interventions. Before proceeding to some of the philosophical problems that arise in this domain, it will help to have some background on evidence in medicine. In this chapter we study some of the fundamental challenges to generating reliable evidence in medicine, and some of the methods that medical researchers use to address these challenges. These methods raise a plethora of philosophical puzzles, which we begin to investigate in this chapter and proceed to investigate in more detail in chapter 9.

Medical research is prone to bias. When evaluating the effectiveness of a medical intervention, a bias is a feature of the design of a study, or the execution of a study, or the analysis of the data from a study, that makes the evidence misleading. In medical research biases tend to generate evidence that suggests that medical interventions are more effective and safer than they in fact are. Researchers respond to concerns about bias by using methodological safeguards. These can be relatively reliable tactics to block the threat from a particular form of bias. In this chapter, we examine some prominent forms of bias in medical research. There are many more. David Sackett, one of the founders of the evidence-based medicine movement, described 56 subtypes of bias in medical research, including volunteer bias, missing clinical data bias, withdrawal bias, compliance bias, bogus control bias, exposure suspicion bias, recall bias, instrument bias, and repeated peeks bias. One of the worst forms of bias in medical research now is publication bias, which we investigate in chapter 8.

The most important method for measuring effectiveness of interventions, at least according to EBM, is the randomized trial. The main feature that distinguishes randomized trials as reliable, according to proponents, is that the allocation of subjects to the experimental and control group of studies is done randomly. But the importance of randomization is debated. Many people hold meta-analyses of RCTs to be the definitive empirical basis of evaluating medical interventions, but this too is controversial. Another research strategy is to supplement findings from population-level studies such as RCTs with knowledge of mechanisms: the microphysiological parts and processes that constitute diseases and the way medical interventions act on those parts and processes. But the importance of mechanisms is also debated. This chapter introduces these debates.

7.2 PHASES OF MEDICAL RESEARCH

Medical research on the effectiveness of interventions is organized into several "phases." Phase 0 refers to "preclinical" research, which is the study of the chemical properties of a pharmaceutical intervention and the effects of that intervention on cell and tissue cultures. This is also the phase in which the experimental intervention is tested on animals. This phase is called preclinical because it is research on an intervention prior to that intervention being tested in human populations in clinics and hospitals.

Phase 1 trials are the first time an experimental intervention is tested in humans. Usually phase 1 trials include very few subjects (from a handful to several dozen people). Researchers look for significant harmful effects of the intervention in phase 1 trials. If the results from a phase 1 trial suggest that the intervention is not excessively harmful, the intervention gets tested in phase 2 trials.

Phase 2 trials include more subjects, roughly around one hundred or so, and are randomized controlled trials (RCTs). A randomized controlled trial (RCT) involves administering an experimental intervention to one group of subjects (the experimental group), administering a placebo or competitor intervention to another group of subjects (the control group), measuring parameters of the subjects, and comparing the values of those parameters between the two groups, and if the average values of parameters differ between groups, inferring that the intervention has a general capacity to cause that difference. Trials usually have methodological safeguards to minimize systematic error, prominently including the random allocation of subjects to groups, and concealment of the group assignment from both the investigators and the subjects.

In phase 2 RCTs researchers continue to hunt for harmful effects of the experimental intervention but also assess the potential beneficial effects of the intervention. If the results from a phase 2 trial appear promising, the intervention gets tested in phase 3 trials. Phase 3 trials are the most important step in evaluating experimental interventions. These are also randomized trials and are larger than phase 2 trials, sometimes including thousands of subjects. These trials can sometimes last several years and be carried out in many countries. Regulatory agencies typically require that multiple phase 3 trials show a positive effect of an intervention in order for that intervention to be approved for general clinical use.

After an intervention has been approved by regulators, any further studies on the intervention are called phase 4 studies (sometimes these are called "post-approval" studies). In some cases phase 4 studies are RCTs. But most phase 4 studies are non-randomized studies, such as case-control studies or cohort studies.

A case-control study involves identifying subjects with a particular feature, like having a particular disease (these subjects are called "cases"), and comparing these cases with other subjects who do not have that feature (these subjects are called "controls"). Typically researchers determine the proportion of cases and controls who have been exposed, in the past, to a particular putative cause of the feature. If the proportion of cases who have been exposed to the putative cause is higher than the proportion of controls who have been exposed to the putative cause, then this is some evidence that the putative cause is a genuine cause of the feature. The main methodological risk of case-control studies is that there might be a confounding factor that increases the probability of a person having both the putative cause and the feature, in which case there would be a spurious correlation between the putative cause and the feature. This is the problem that randomization is meant to mitigate (we will ask whether or not randomization is successful at this in §7.5).

7.3 BIAS

One of the most pervasive forms of bias is called "confirmation bias." People give more weight to evidence that confirms their pre-evidence beliefs and less weight to evidence that disconfirms their pre-evidence beliefs. If a person uses a drug to treat a disease, that person (and their physicians, friends, and family) will tend to interpret his subsequent improvement as being caused by the drug, whether or not such improvement was actually caused by the drug. Confirmation bias is confounded by the placebo effect, in which consumers of medical interventions report improvements in their health merely as a result of receiving some form of treatment—the mere consumption of a medical intervention generates an expectation of improvement, and the expectation then gets multiplied by confirmation bias.

Confirmation bias is further exacerbated by the natural course of diseases. Suppose the severity of symptoms of a disease fluctuates over time (like bipolar disorder), so that there are more severe periods and less severe periods. If a person seeks treatment during a more severe period, the severity of her symptoms will decrease after intervention, regardless of the effectiveness of the treatment. If the severity of symptoms of a disease decreases over time (as with most cases of the common cold), then the same consideration applies: the severity of symptoms will decrease after intervention, whether or not that intervention contributed to the decrease in symptoms. In both of these cases it is merely the passage of time that causes the alleviation of symptoms. For all of the above reasons, single-case reports about a patient's experiences with a medical intervention should be interpreted with great caution.

In the context of medical research, confirmation bias has been mitigated by methodological safeguards. These include testing the intervention in multiple subjects and using control groups, which allows for an assessment of the effectiveness of an intervention despite the natural course of an illness. Another safeguard involves concealment of which groups (intervention or control) subjects are allocated to, which is also called "blinding" (this decreases the expectation of improvement, since ideally subjects do not know if they are in the control group or not). The use of placebos is an attempt to ensure that subjects do not guess what group they are in—though what exactly a placebo is has been a matter of debate. The very idea of a placebo raises the question about what the basic aims of medicine are, and whether or not placebos can be considered effective medical interventions (we will examine such questions in chapter 10).

These safeguards do not always work. It is common for subjects and their treating physicians to accurately guess what group they are in, on the basis of their responses to the intervention that they have been assigned—in such cases, the blinding is broken. Outside the context of controlled medical research there are no such safeguards, and most people reason in ways that are influenced by confirmation bias: people regularly attribute improvements in their health to medical interventions that they have recently used.

Another widespread form of bias in medical research is called "design bias." Medical studies that employ some of the safeguards noted above can nevertheless have design features, often quite subtle properties of a study, that render the study biased. A design bias is a bias built into the internal design of a research method.

A widespread type of design bias is called selection bias. One of the basic elements of medical research, as noted above, is to compare subjects in an intervention group with subjects in a control group. If there is a measured difference in the outcomes between the two groups, we might infer that it was the intervention that caused the difference. To reliably infer this, the subjects in the two groups must be similar with respect to all the other possible factors that could influence the outcome. Selection bias is when there is a relevant difference between the subjects in the two groups.

Randomizing the allocation of subjects into groups is an attempt to avoid selection bias by taking the allocation of subjects out of the control of researchers. Below we examine an argument that concludes that randomization does not guarantee that subjects in the two groups will be similar in all salient respects, but the hope is that randomization will at least minimize such differences. Selection bias is especially worrying for non-randomized studies such as case-control studies; however, critics argue that even trials that employ randomization to avoid selection bias can still suffer from that very bias because real trials are not ideal trials (§7.5).

Another example of design bias is called "instrument bias." This occurs when the measuring instruments employed in a clinical trial are tuned in such a way that a medical intervention appears more effective and safer than it truly is. Here is an example of instrument bias from toxicology, in which the problem had to do with the choice of animal model (the "instrument" in this case is the animal). Bisphenol A (BPA) is used in some plastic products and is suspected of causing cancer and other harmful effects, due to its similarity to estrogen. Most of the studies testing the harms of BPA in rats that were performed by non-industry scientists found harmful effects of BPA, but none of the studies funded by industry did so. The problem was that industry studies used strains of rats that were less sensitive to estrogen.

The analysis of data from trials can be biased. One way this can occur is when researchers analyze their data in multiple unconstrained ways to look for differences between the experimental group and the control group. A trial can make many different kinds of measurements, the data can be sorted in many ways (for example, subjects' ages can be measured to the day, but can then be grouped in an infinite number of ways), and many statistical tests can be applied to a single set of data. This practice is known as "p-hacking." P-hacking increases the chance that researchers will find spurious signals in their data.

A related form of design bias is a result of the many subjective decisions that must be made by researchers when analyzing their data, including how missing data and outlying data are handled, how skewed data is treated (for instance, sometimes skewed data is transformed into a "normal" distribution because some analyses require normal distributions). Analysts have a lot of freedom when making such choices, and every unconstrained decision permits more possible analyses with more potential for generating spurious results.

One way that medical science attempts to mitigate this problem of unconstrained analysis or researcher degrees of freedom is to require researchers to plan their analysis in advance of a trial, and to publish the plan so that others can assess the extent of such bias. Unfortunately some empirical evaluations suggest that despite the pre-publication of analysis plans, medical scientists very often depart from such plans.

7.4 ANIMAL MODELS

To help determine whether an experimental intervention will be safe for humans, and to determine the right dosing for humans, medical scientists perform experiments on animals. In order to use an animal to get evidence that is relevant to evaluating the effectiveness and safety of an intervention for humans, researchers need an "animal model" of the disease in question. An animal model of a human disease is a disease in an animal that is as similar as possible to the human disease in its pathophysiology and symptoms. For some diseases this is straightforward, but for other diseases, especially for psychiatric diseases, it is difficult to develop an animal model of diseases. The use of animals in medical research is a difficult ethical problem, but here we focus on the pertinent epistemological problems.

A good example of using animal models in medical research is the discovery by Banting and Best that type 1 diabetes is caused by an insulin deficiency. They blocked the function of the pancreases of dogs in various ways (either by removing the pancreases or by ligating them), and observed that the dogs developed symptoms of diabetes. Thus, Banting and Best were able to develop a canine model of diabetes. They then extracted a substance from the pancreas of dogs and cows, and this substance was able to reverse the symptoms of diabetes in the dogs that had their pancreatic function blocked. They isolated and purified this substance and called it insulin. This was a profoundly important discovery. Insulin is extremely effective for treating humans with diabetes.

Unfortunately, the use of animal models to provide evidence that is relevant to causal inferences for humans is far from straightforward. One obvious concern about animal models is the extent to which animal physiology is similar to human physiology. The question is this: Are we justified in extrapolating results from animal models to humans? If an intervention does x in animals, can we expect it to do x in humans? In some cases, like the canine models that Banting and Best used, there is sufficient similarity between animals and humans such that extrapolation is warranted. But in other cases the similarity is less clear. Could we have a reliable animal model of depression, for example? What are the conditions under which an extrapolation from animals to humans is warranted?

Suppose that in carefully controlled experiments, researchers find that a particular chemical, which is widely used in manufacturing consumer products, causes cancer in rodents. Obviously we want to know if this chemical causes cancer in humans. But we cannot go through all the phases of medical research described in §7.2, because it would be unethical to intentionally administer this chemical to humans, given the possibility that it can cause cancer. The evidence from rodents might be the best evidence we can get.

The general form of an extrapolative inference is this:

Extrapolative Inference: Since we have evidence that d causes x in a base population, d causes x in a target population.

Notice that this is a very general formulation of extrapolation—it applies to all extrapolative inferences, and not just from animals to humans. For example, suppose we find that d causes x in a phase 3 randomized trial. Can we infer that d causes x in the general human population? This is a question about extrapolation.

Notice also that extrapolation is fundamentally an inductive inference—the formulation of extrapolation can be reiterated in a more general way as this: since we have evidence that d causes x in this spatiotemporal context, d causes x in that spatiotemporal context. This latter formulation is just a general statement of induction. However, we will not worry about general philosophical concerns about induction here, and instead focus on the more specific concerns raised by extrapolation from animal models to humans (we examine extrapolation from one human population to another in chapter 9).

Is extrapolation warranted? How should researchers go about extrapolating? Let's examine three views regarding extrapolation: simple extrapolation, strict extrapolation, and mechanism-based extrapolation.

Here is one easy answer to the question about the justification of extrapolation: always presume that extrapolative inference is justified. In other words, if one finds that d causes x in a base population, one can always infer that d causes x in a target population. So if a chemical causes cancer in rodents, we can infer that this chemical causes cancer in humans. This is "simple extrapolation." As we will see in chapter 9, simple extrapolation from one human population to another is assumed to be justified by evidence-based medicine. Simple extrapolation can be made slightly more sophisticated by noting similarities between the base population and the target population, such as one would find based on phylogenetic proximity—for instance, one could say that simple induction is fine when the base population and the target population are evolutionarily close (say, from rodents to humans), but not when the two populations are evolutionarily distant (say, from flies to humans).

The problem with simple extrapolation is that it is too simple: it leads to many false conclusions about causal relations in target populations. Critics raise two thorny challenges for extrapolation. The first is called the "extrapolator's circle." As noted above, extrapolation relies on relevant similarities between the base population (in this case, animals) and the target population (humans). The necessary kinds of similarities typically require knowing a great deal about the physiological mechanisms of both the base population *and* the target population. The extrapolator's circle is the challenge of knowing that the physiological mechanisms of the target population are sufficiently similar to the physiological mechanisms of the base population *without* already knowing about the causal relation in the target population that we are making an extrapolative inference about.

Here's another way to put the problem. To infer that d causes x in the target population from the fact that d caused x in the base population, we need to know that the base population and the target population are similar in relevant respects. Which respects? One answer is this: all those respects that allow d to cause x. However, to know that much about the target population, we either would already have enough knowledge to infer that d causes x in the target population, or we would already have inferred that d causes x in the target population. If the former, then we have no need for extrapolation in the first place, and if the latter, then we are stuck in a vicious circle, since to extrapolate that d causes x in the target population we would have had to extrapolate that d causes x in the target population.

The second challenge for extrapolation from animals to humans is the variability of physiological mechanisms in different species: how can extrapolation from one species to another be justified if we know that physiological mechanisms differ from one species to another?

Some critics of animal research have emphasized these concerns about simple extrapolation, and propose instead a view that we can call "strict extrapolation," which holds that only if there are no causally relevant differences between a target and base population, then, if d causes x in the base population, infer that d causes x in the target population. That is, strict extrapolation holds, as a necessary condition, that the target population and base population have no causally relevant differences.

The problem with strict extrapolation is that it is too strict: there are always causally relevant differences between species, and there are even such differences between members of the same species. Thus, strict extrapolation leads to many missed opportunities for making reliable inferences about causal relations in target populations. Notice that strict extrapolation also faces the extrapolator's circle. If we are required to know the exact causal mechanism linking d to x in both the base population and the target population before we are permitted to extrapolate from the former to the latter, then, in virtue of the fact that we know the causal mechanism linking d to x in the target population, we do not need to extrapolate after all (since we would already know that d causes x in the target population).

Mechanism-based extrapolation is a middle-ground position between simple extrapolation and strict extrapolation. The basic idea is to determine the extent of similarities and differences between physiological mechanisms of a base population and target population. As above, one source of evidence that pertains to assessing such similarities could be phylogenetic relatedness. But researchers can also study the similarities and differences between the relevant physiological mechanisms with a variety of empirical means. To avoid the problems with simple and strict extrapolation, mechanism-based extrapolation starts by describing a course-grained schema of the mechanism linking d to x, and then discovers the specific parts and processes that constitute the mechanism, often by tracing the causal pathways backward and forward from particular parts of the mechanism. Extrapolation can be justified if we know the mechanism linking d to x in the base population, and then we compare parts and processes of the mechanism in the target population to the mechanism in the base population and focus on the parts and processes that are most likely to be relevantly different. (Daniel Steel calls this "comparative process tracing.") The more similar the mechanisms are, the more justified extrapolation is.

To illustrate, suppose that in the base population d causes x, via the mechanism $d{\to}A{\to}B{\to}C{\to}D{\to}E{\to}x$. Does d cause x in the target population? Suppose we know that in the target population, C→D. We then examine the other parts of the mechanism, forward and backward. We also have very good reason to believe that in the target population d→A and B→C, so we don't need to examine those stages of the mechanism. We focus on the other stages, and we confirm that in the target population, A→B, D→E, and E→x. We can thus extrapolate that in the target population, d causes x. This is a mechanism-based extrapolation.

This method can take into account nuances such as situations in which the mechanisms are highly similar except for a single salient difference that completely undermines the extrapolation. Does this method solve the challenges to the other views about extrapolation? Mechanism-based extrapolation still requires knowing a lot about the physiological mechanisms of both the base population and the target population, and so critics of strict extrapolation can criticize mechanism-based extrapolation on this ground as well. Moreover, we often know very little about the relevant mechanism in either the base population or the target population. Without very detailed knowledge about the mechanism in the base population and the mechanism in the target population, mechanism-based extrapolation can be misleading. In the schematic example above, for instance, the target population could share the exact same mechanism that links d to x as the base population, yet have an additional inhibitory pathway from E to x such that d no longer causes x (say, E→P→~x). We will return to the subject of mechanism-based causal inferences in §7.7.

Animals have been used for researching many diseases, but it is especially difficult to develop animal models of psychiatric diseases. This is in part because we understand so little about the pathophysiology of most psychiatric diseases (see chapter 12). It is also because most psychiatric diseases are defined with reference to behavioral patterns, emotions, and intentional states that are fundamentally human, such as the enjoyment of one's hobbies, and animal models can at best be distant analogues of such human features. Interpreting animal models with respect to human mental traits is fraught with uncertainty. For example, the "Morris water navigation task" (sometimes called the "Morris water maze") is an experimental set-up in which rodents are placed in tanks of water, and then the rodents are timed to see how long it takes them to escape the tank. The factors that influence escape time, such as age, can then be studied. However, the mental phenomena that such escape time is meant to provide evidence about is underdetermined: some say it is spatial navigation, some say it is the development of cognitive maps, some say it is simply a behavioral change.

7.5 RANDOMIZATION

Randomized controlled trials (RCTs) have become central to testing the effectiveness of medical interventions. The first randomized studies were used to test alleged psychic phenomena in the beginning of the twentieth century: researchers studying psychic phenomena kept getting evidence of various sorts of psychic effects, but when randomizing techniques were introduced into their studies such phenomena disappeared. Thus randomization was used as a debunking methodology. Randomized trials continued to serve that function as they became more common in the second half of the twentieth century in medical research.

Those in the evidence-based medicine (EBM) movement, which became prominent toward the end of the twentieth century, hold that medical interventions must be tested with randomized trials. All other forms of evidence, according to EBM—including evidence from non-randomized population studies (for example, cohort studies) and evidence of mechanisms—are unreliable and should be ignored. To illustrate this epistemological stance, EBM developed "evidence hierarchies," described above. Here is an exemplary passage from leaders in EBM:

> Evidence-based medicine de-emphasizes intuition, unsystematic clinical experience, and pathophysiological rationale as sufficient grounds for clinical decision making and stresses the examination of evidence from clinical research (Guyatt et al. 1992).

A variety of arguments have been proposed to justify the importance of randomized trials. One is similar to the story about psychic phenomena: EBM scientists claim that randomized trials have been used to debunk many medical interventions that were thought to be effective but upon testing with randomized trials turned out to be ineffective. Let's call this the *debunking argument*. Another argument is based on a concern about confounding factors. We saw this worry earlier, when learning about selection bias (§7.3): if the subjects in the intervention group and control group of a study differ with respect to a certain factor, call it Z, and Z itself influences the measured outcome in the study, then if there is a measured difference in the outcome between the two groups, that difference might be due not to the intervention but rather to Z. Z could be the age of subjects, say (younger subjects typically fare better in trials than older subjects), or the background health status of subjects, or how affected by placebos they are. The virtue of randomization, many claim, is that it guarantees that Z is balanced between the two groups. Let's call this the *balance argument*.

Each of these arguments in favor of randomization has been challenged by critics. In response to the debunking argument, note that a premise of the argument is that non-randomized studies overestimate the effectiveness of interventions while randomized trials accurately estimate the effectiveness of interventions. While this might be true in some cases, for some interventions, it is not generally true. Randomized trials have many design features that render them likely to overestimate the effectiveness of interventions. There have been recent empirical assessments of the relative assessments of effectiveness between randomized and non-randomized studies, and there appears to be little difference in their tendencies to over- or underestimate effectiveness.

In response to the balance argument, critics claim that a single act of randomization could still leave the two study groups imbalanced on a confounding factor (a Z), on the basis of chance alone. Imagine you have a pocket full of coins. You take each coin out of your pocket, flip it, and put the coins that land heads in one pile and those that land tails in another pile. Would you be surprised if the two piles were of slightly different sizes? Of course, the more coins you flip the closer the two piles will be in size, but you have a finite number of coins, and hence no matter how many coins you flip, the two piles are likely to be different sizes. Similarly in randomized trials. If a trial randomly allocates ten subjects to each group, then for every Z there is a chance that it will be imbalanced. And there are many, many possible Zs: some we know about, and some we don't. Since no trial has infinitely many subjects, there is little reason to think that a randomized trial in fact balances all the potential confounding factors.

There are many other worries about randomized trials. One worry is based on how subjects are recruited to trials: most trials employ inclusion and exclusion criteria that serve to control for the kinds of people who are subjects in trials. For example, trials often exclude old people, women, people on multiple drugs, and people with other diseases, and these are the sorts of people who will go on to use the intervention if it gets approved. This entails a concern about extrapolating from the results of trials to expectations about how effective an intervention will be in the clinical "real world" setting. Another worry about trials is their duration: many trials are very short, just long enough to detect a short-term beneficial effect of an intervention, but not long enough to determine whether the effect is sustained over the long run or to determine whether the intervention has harmful effects that are caused in the longer-run.

Many scientists, physicians, and regulators believe that randomized trials provide a definitive evidential basis for assessing the effectiveness of medical interventions. Indeed, many hold that randomized trials are both necessary and sufficient for confirming or disconfirming hypotheses regarding the effectiveness of medical interventions. But the above problems show that randomized trials *simpliciter* cannot be sufficient to justify causal hypotheses (because there are all sorts of ways in which the evidence from a trial might be misleading).

Consider a fun example. A researcher tested the effects of retroactive, intercessory prayer—praying on behalf of others in retrospect, years after the outcome that was measured—to see whether it could improve outcomes for hospitalized patients (Leibovici 2001). He examined all patients who had been admitted to a particular hospital from 1990 to 1996 for bloodstream infections. In the year 2000, he randomly allocated some of those patients to an intervention group and some to a control group. He checked the two groups for imbalances in potential confounds, and found none. Those in the intervention group received "a short prayer for the well being and full recovery of the group as a whole." In other words, the intervention group was being prayed for in retrospect—they had been in the hospital anywhere from four to ten years before the trial. Then the medical records were examined, and Leibovici found that mortality in the prayed-for group was 28.1%, and in the control group it was 30.2% (which was not quite statistically significant), and the duration of stay in the hospital and duration of fever were shorter in the prayed-for group (and this was statistically significant). The study was not intended to be taken seriously as research but was meant to be a satirical demonstration of the fallibility of randomized trials (we will see in chapter 9 that the example also illustrates a more fundamental issue regarding scientific inference).

Moreover, critics argue that randomization is not necessary in order for a study to provide compelling evidence for or against a causal hypothesis. In one sense this is obvious because science discovered causal relations for a very long time without randomized trials. Consider another fun example. We think parachutes are effective interventions for slowing one's fall out of an airplane. Indeed, most of us are convinced of their effectiveness for slowing one's fall. But parachutes have never been tested by an RCT! The very idea is absurd, and the reason it is absurd is that most of us are already convinced of their effectiveness, regardless of the lack of evidence from randomized trials. In §7.7 we will learn about mechanistic reasoning for causal hypotheses—one reason for our justified confidence in the effectiveness of parachutes, in addition to our historical experience with them, is that we know exactly how they work because we carefully designed them.

7.6 META-ANALYSIS

The technique called "meta-analysis" involves amalgamating the outcome measures from multiple studies into one overall outcome measure. This can be valuable because often the primary studies are too small and so their outcome measures are unreliable, but if multiple outcome measures from multiple studies are amalgamated then the larger size of the combined outcome measure can be more reliable. For this reason meta-analyses of randomized trials are typically thought to be the best form of evidence for assessing the effectiveness of medical interventions. Indeed, some of the major organizations in evidence-based medicine, such as the Cochrane Collaboration, primarily use meta-analysis.

There is a strange thing about meta-analysis, however. Multiple meta-analyses based on the same primary evidence can reach contradictory conclusions. For example, in 2005 two meta-analyses were published in the same issue of the *British Medical Journal*, asking whether the use of selective serotonin reuptake inhibitors (SSRIs, a class of antidepressants) increases the chance of attempting suicide. One found no link between SSRI use and suicide attempts, while another found a link between SSRI use and suicide attempts. (The two meta-analyses were Gunnell, Saperia, and Ashby 2005 and Fergusson et al. 2005.) How can this be? If multiple meta-analyses on the very same hypothesis, based on the same evidence, can reach contradictory conclusions, can meta-analysis be trusted?

The reason that multiple meta-analyses can reach contradictory conclusions is that, just like trials, the technique involves numerous unconstrained choices. These include which primary evidence to include in the first place (all available evidence? only randomized trials? only randomized trials of a certain size or quality?), which quantitative analyses to use, and which method of assessing trial quality to use. Different decisions on these methodological choices can lead to different outcomes.

But aren't all scientific methods like that? Indeed, many or most scientific methods are sensitive to fine-grained methodological choices. Attempts to detect high-energy physical particles, preparing cell cultures to be viewed under a microscope, or using the red-shift of galaxies to measure the rate of expansion of the universe—all these techniques require particular methodological choices. So, sensitivity to methodological choices itself cannot be a mark against a scientific method, including meta-analysis. But often scientists can develop reasoned arguments for one methodological choice over another, and sometimes a technique simply will not give any result if the right choices are not made. In the case of meta-analysis, some of the required choices are such that there is no right or wrong approach—the decisions are fundamentally arbitrary—and thus reasoned arguments can't be offered for some choices in meta-analysis. However, for other choices in meta-analysis there are better ways to carry out the method. For example, some meta-analyses are able to get access to all data from randomized trials even if that data hadn't been published—this approach is able to overcome the pernicious problem of publication bias (discussed in chapter 8) and thereby give more reliable results.

There are two further reasons for concern about meta-analysis. One is about the quality of the primary evidence that is amalgamated by meta-analysis. We saw above that randomized trials can have a number of problems, and meta-analysis does not necessarily wash these problems away, but rather it inherits the problems (this is called the "garbage-in-garbage-out" argument against meta-analysis). Another shortcoming of meta-analysis is that it ignores a wide range of pertinent evidence. By its very nature meta-analysis is able to include only particular kinds of quantitative evidence. But many people argue that other forms of evidence are crucially important for assessing the effectiveness of medical interventions, including mechanistic evidence. We turn to this in the next section.

7.7 MECHANISMS

The term "mechanism" has taken on a technical meaning in philosophy of science in recent years. Mechanisms are roughly defined as a collection of entities and their activities that work together to generate particular kinds of outputs from particular inputs. The notion of mechanism is especially pertinent to biological and medical sciences, since these are domains in which the objects of study are often complicated arrangements of microphysiological parts and their interactions.

In the epistemology of medical research there are two radical views regarding the role of mechanisms in causal inference (and specifically in assessing the effectiveness of medical interventions), and a middle-ground view that sits somewhere between the radical views.

One radical view, which is often expressed by leaders in EBM, is the *black box* thesis. The black box thesis holds that causal inference in medicine should be based only on the quantitative summaries of randomized trials or other population-level studies (I'll call this kind of evidence "statistical evidence"). If evidence from trials says that drug d does x, then black boxers say that we should believe that d does x. This view is called the black box thesis because it holds that we should consider the mechanistic basis of diseases and interventions as "black boxes" that do not need to be understood in order to believe that d does x.

The opposing radical view is the *mechanista* thesis. The mechanista thesis holds that causal inference in medicine must be based in part on mechanistic evidence. The term *mechanistic evidence* is shorthand for inferences based on reasoning from knowledge of mechanisms to expected effects of interventions. Mechanistas hold that statistical evidence is insufficient to warrant causal inferences about interventions, and that both mechanistic and statistical evidence are necessary. Some mechanistas also hold that mechanistic evidence alone can be sufficient to warrant causal inferences about interventions. If evidence from trials says that d does x, and we have no mechanistic evidence about d, then mechanistas hold that we ought not believe that d does x. Some mechanistas hold that if we have mechanistic evidence that d does x, that is sufficient to believe that d does x, even in the absence of statistical evidence for the causal relation.

A middle view is the *pluralist* thesis, which holds that neither statistical evidence nor mechanistic evidence is necessary for causal inference, though knowledge of mechanisms can sometimes or often be helpful in warranting causal inferences. A famous example of a medical scientist who held this view was Sir Bradford Hill, who argued that there are a variety of sorts of evidence that can be appealed to when assessing causal hypotheses in medicine, none of which are necessary but all of which can be helpful (§9.2). Older terms for these competing views harken back to traditional debates in epistemology: *rationalism* about causal inferences in medicine is the corresponding older term for the mechanista thesis, and *empiricism* about causal inferences in medicine is the corresponding older term for the black box thesis.

There is a seductive, straightforward argument for the black box thesis: if the evidence from our most reliable studies suggests that d does x, then what else do we have to base our judgment on whether or not d does x? The most responsible thing for us to believe is that d does x; that is what the evidence says, and we should believe the evidence. Let's call this the *evidence-based argument* for the black box thesis. For example, in 1753 when Lind found that eating citrus fruits could help treat scurvy, scientists had no knowledge whatsoever regarding how citrus fruits could do this. The very idea of a vitamin deficiency was impossible, because vitamins hadn't been discovered yet. But giving citrus juice to people with scurvy was still an effective intervention.

Another argument in favor of the black box thesis is that our knowledge of mechanisms is often incomplete and can lead us astray. This is especially the case when mechanistic reasoning is based on faulty physiological theories. To take an extreme example, under humoral theory psychosis was thought to be the result of an excess of blood and yellow bile, and thus, based on mechanistic reasoning, a standard treatment for psychosis was bloodletting. There are many contemporary examples of this (interested readers could investigate antiarrhythmic drugs, hormone-replacement therapy for menopausal women, or rofecoxib, as examples). Let's call this the *trouble-in-the-box argument* for the black box thesis.

There is a seductive, straightforward argument for the mechanista thesis: if we know *how* an intervention works, then it follows that we know *that* an intervention works, and thus we can justify causal inferences about medical interventions by appealing to how interventions operate in disease pathophysiology. Let's call this the *know-how argument*. Recall the parachute example: we know how parachutes work, and it would be absurd, when testing the effectiveness of parachutes to slow one's falling from an airplane, to demand a population-level study comparing parachute-wearers to a control group of non-parachute-wearers.

Another argument in favor of the mechanista thesis is that statistical evidence is often misleading and can lead us astray. Think back to the various forms of bias discussed in §7.3, and the problems with trials noted in §7.5. Statistical evidence is fallible, says the mechanista, so when using statistical evidence to warrant causal inferences about medical interventions, such evidence should be supplemented with mechanistic evidence. Let's call this the *trouble-in-the-data argument* for the mechanista thesis. A good example is the study described in §7.5 about retroactive intercessory prayer.

Notice that the know-how argument is the flip-side of the trouble-in-the-box argument, and that the trouble-in-the-data argument is the flip-side of the evidence-based argument. This suggests that both sides are too strong, and motivates the pluralist thesis. Sometimes statistical evidence alone is sufficient to warrant causal inferences about medical interventions, but reasoning about medical interventions by appealing to both statistical and mechanistic evidence is the safest way to make such inferences.

However, there is a third and more general argument in favor of the mechanista thesis. Whenever one makes an inference one should base the inference not only on one's recently acquired evidence, but also on one's background beliefs and other forms of evidence and relevant theories. In the case of inferences about medical interventions, such background knowledge can include any mechanistic evidence that one has about that intervention. This very general norm of inference is explained in chapter 9. For now, note that the black box thesis violates this norm.

FURTHER READING

Randomization: Urbach (1985), Worrall (2002), Hacking (1988), Cartwright (2010)
Evidence-based medicine: Upshur (2002), Goldenberg, Borgerson, and Bluhm (2009), Howick (2011b)
Bias: Rawlins (2008), Sackett (1979)
Animal models and extrapolation: Steel (2007), LaFollette and Shanks (1996), Weber (2005), Sullivan (2010)
Meta-analysis: Stegenga (2011), Jukola (2015)
Mechanisms: Clarke, Gillies, Illari, Russo and Williamson (2014), Howick (2011a), Leuridan and Weber (2011), Illari (2011), Tulodziecki (2013)

1. Is knowledge of the mechanism by which an intervention works necessary and/or sufficient for making an inference about the effectiveness of that intervention?
2. Can we make reliable inferences regarding the effectiveness and harmfulness of medical interventions with animal research?
3. Describe some of the most worrying threats to the reliability of medical research. How do medical scientists attempt to mitigate those threats? Are those tactics successful?
4. Is meta-analysis the best method for testing the effectiveness of medical interventions?

8 : OBJECTIVITY AND
THE SOCIAL STRUCTURE
OF SCIENCE

8.1 SUMMARY

We saw in chapter 7 that medical research employs a number of methodological safeguards in an attempt to minimize the threat of bias. The hope is that such methods render medical research objective. What is objectivity? Is medical research objective?

The terms *objective* and *objectivity* have multiple meanings in science, though one way or another they all amount to terms of praise. In science, objectivity can be a term that applies to research methods, or to the evidence generated by such methods (or sometimes, to scientists themselves). Objectivity of a research method pertains to the extent to which that method is free from systematic bias. We could just as well use the term *reliable*. Objectivity of evidence pertains to the extent to which evidence is reliable for making inferences, or the extent to which evidence is truth-conducive: the more that evidence is objective, the more it is an unbiased guide to the truth. Objectivity can also be a property that applies to the community-level of science: a scientific community can be organized and act in ways that are more or less conducive to the discovery of truth.

We saw some ways that research methods in medicine can be biased in chapter 7. The focus there was on possible errors generated by the research methods themselves. Here the focus is on "social objectivity"—the possible biases that arise due to shortcomings in the social structure of the scientific community, and the various ways that the community structure of medical science can mitigate such biases and thereby achieve a degree of objectivity.

Publication bias and conflicts of interest that arise due to industry funding of medical research are two hugely important problems in medicine today, so we start the chapter with discussions of these problems. After a brief look at the classic demarcation problem, we turn to another general topic that has become prominent in philosophy of science: the influence of values in scientific research. The influence of values on medical science is, arguably, a threat to its objectivity. One possible resolution is to try to mitigate these threats by implementing epistemological tactics at the social level.

8.2 INDUSTRY FUNDING AND PUBLICATION BIAS

Once a medical study is complete, the researchers must choose what to do with the evidence from the study. The standard practice is to publish the results in a medical journal. However, evidence that suggests that a medical intervention is ineffective is less likely to be published than evidence that suggests that a medical intervention is effective. This phenomenon is known as publication bias and is widespread in medicine. A related problem is reporting bias. This occurs when researchers do publish the results of a trial, but publish only some of the evidence (usually, that which suggests the drug is effective). Reporting bias and publication bias are problems with medical research that transcend the methods themselves.

Publication bias occurs at all phases of clinical research. Examples of publication bias are easy to find. Here is a striking example. A German health technology assessment agency started with all of the drugs that had been submitted to the agency, and went back to the submitted trial designs for these drugs and counted the number of measured outcomes in these trials, and then counted the number of measured outcomes for these trials that appeared in publications. Less than one quarter of all outcomes that had been measured had been published.

Of course, in science generally there is a tendency toward not publishing "null" findings—results of studies that are not "statistically significant," or results of studies that are not indicative of an interesting phenomenon. In chapter 9 we will study problems with the standard of statistical significance, which is a central notion of frequentist statistics. What counts as an "interesting" finding is highly context dependent. In the context of clinical research, in which medical interventions are being tested for effectiveness and safety, arguably the evidence is always important to know about.

Industry sponsors of medical research claim that because they paid for a study, they own the evidence from that study and can freely choose to publish it or not. Critics of this claim that when it comes to medical interventions, all evidence should be publicly available as a matter of basic rights. This raises other thorny questions about the role of private industry versus governments in testing medical interventions.

Biases in medical research can be rendered more serious by conflicts of interest. Conflicts of interest in medicine are widespread: they exist among industrial manufacturers of medical interventions, researchers, regulators, clinical guideline writers, patient advocacy groups, medical teachers and authors of textbooks, and even scholarly journals. The most important form of conflict of interest arises from financial relations. In this section we study several examples of conflicts of interest in medical research and regulation to illustrate how significant the problem is.

Medical researchers and physicians are usually employed by universities and hospitals, but in addition to their regular jobs, many hold positions in companies that sponsor research, own shares of corporations that manufacture medical interventions, receive payments for consulting with industry, own patents that are licensed to industry, and receive fees for enrolling their patients in trials.

Conflicts of interest are present not just among individual researchers but also among institutions. An obvious form of this is the financial incentive for companies to demonstrate that one of their products is effective. Most clinical trials of medical interventions are funded by the manufacturers of the very interventions being evaluated. Even medical journals can have conflicts of interest because many journals receive a large portion of their budgets from advertisements paid for by manufacturers of the products that are evaluated in articles published in those journals. Financial conflicts of interest exist in regulatory agencies. The FDA relies on advisory committees, and many members of these committees have financial interests in the products being evaluated by the committees.

There are two strategies that are employed by journals, regulators, and universities to mitigate the influence of financial conflicts of interest. One is to constrain the severity of conflicts of interest. For example, financial relationships can be capped at certain values. Some universities limit the amount that their staff can receive from private companies, for instance. Another strategy is to require the disclosure of conflicts of interest. For example, when journals use this strategy, they require that articles published in the journals include information about the author's relevant financial ties. Many granting agencies and journals require scientists to disclose the various sources of funds they have received from private companies.

It is a platitude that these tactics are useful for mitigating the influence of conflicts of interest on bias in research. But critics claim that these tactics are not sufficient. A stronger tactic would be full prohibition of conflicts of interest, enforced by universities, professional societies, journals, or more powerful institutions. A rejoinder against this, some argue, is that full prohibition of conflicts of interest would lead to the slowing of scientific progress; for example, if a journal prohibited conflicts of interest, some claim, then scientists might be deterred from publishing. However, this empirical claim about the motives of scientists is dubious—scientists have typically sought to publish their work for motives other than financial reasons, such as a desire to share their work in a communal enterprise of discovery, or a desire for credit. An even stronger strategy would be to altogether eliminate financial incentives in medical research, by a variety of means such as eliminating intellectual property protection—I discuss this more controversial idea in chapter 13.

You might wish for a more principled and more general solution to the above concerns about bias in research. Such a motivation is especially pressing for medical research. One possible approach could be to develop norms for demarcating legitimate from illegitimate scientific activity. The general version of this idea is called the "demarcation problem," which has long been a topic for philosophy of science. In the following sections we study various versions of the demarcation problem and attempts to address the problem.

8.3 DEMARCATION

One of the long-standing aims in philosophy of science is to develop a principle that could distinguish good science from bad science (or pseudoscience). Karl Popper's principle of falsificationism is perhaps the best-known attempt to solve the demarcation problem. According to Popper, good science proposes bold theories that can possibly be refuted (or falsified), and rigorous attempts to experimentally or observationally refute such theories must be made; if a falsifiable theory survives attempts at refutation then we ought to maintain a tentative though noncommitted epistemic attitude toward the theory; if the theory is refuted by an observation then it is rejected. Popper's hope was that the principle could be used to demarcate entire disciplines (say, to distinguish astronomy as proper science and astrology as pseudoscience), or to demarcate particular theoretical approaches (say, to distinguish Einstein's theory of relativity as properly scientific from Freud's theory of the ego as pseudoscientific). One reason Popper developed this principle is that he did not believe in inductive theories of scientific confirmation (such as Bayesianism, discussed in chapter 9), and so he needed an alternative theory of inference that did not rely on induction.

Popper's principle of falsificationism has been rejected by philosophers (though its popularity among scientists somehow lingers). Consider some nuanced difficulties. Suppose we are interested in a hypothesis (H) that a new drug is effective at decreasing symptoms of depression. Is H falsifiable? We test H with a randomized trial and find no difference between depressive symptoms in the intervention group compared with the placebo group. Is H falsified? Are trials rigorous enough attempts to refute hypotheses? A defender of the drug could respond by saying that the trial did not last long enough to show improvement of symptoms. So trials cannot be said to be rigorous enough or not, in general, and a particular bit of evidence alone cannot falsify a hypothesis because a defender of the hypothesis can find a way to defend it from an alleged refutation (this problem is an instance of a general problem called "confirmation holism" about scientific inference).

An equally challenging problem for falsificationism is its aversion to statistical models of scientific inference. Consider two hypotheses: drug x lowers blood pressure (H1) and drug y lowers blood pressure (H2). H1 and H2 are equally falsifiable. But H1 has been tested by many randomized trials, and the results suggest that x is in fact effective in lowering blood pressure. H2, on the other hand, has never been tested. Which drug should a patient with high blood pressure take? The evidence supports drug x over drug y. In order to make sense of that claim, we need to rely on a notion of inductive support. But falsificationism denies that such a notion makes sense. So much the worse for falsificationism.

Philosophers have proposed other principles to solve the demarcation problem, but most now believe that attempts to demarcate entire disciplines, or theories, or methods, are misguided. When we consider nuanced details of particular cases, it seems clear that various disciplines or theories or methods can be more-or-less "scientific" or reliable or truth-conducive. Philosophers have adopted the term *objectivity* for the various ways that science can be more-or-less conducive to truth. Moreover, some compelling theories of objectivity hold that the target of evaluation should be a community of science, as opposed to traditional theories of demarcation that hold that it is the work of individual scientists that is assessed by theories of objectivity (such as a view that holds that falsifiability is a property that applies to the theoretical work of a particular scientist). This approach to objectivity will help to assess the extent to which medical research is objective.

8.4 VALUE-LADEN SCIENCE

The above discussion about biases and industry funding of medical research suggests that there is a pernicious influence of non-epistemic values, such as the profit motive of industry, on medical science. A simple solution to this problem would be to prohibit the influence of non-epistemic values in scientific reasoning. Recently, though, many philosophers of science have argued that this is impossible. Seeing why this is the case provides insight into an important aspect of the extent to which medical science can be objective. This, in turn, raises a new kind of demarcation problem.

Let's clear up some terminology. Epistemic values are widely recognized as being important in scientific reasoning—these are features of theories like simplicity and coherence and scope. Simpler theories are said to be better or more likely to be true than complex theories, and the role that simplicity of theories plays in this claim is as an epistemic value. Non-epistemic values are all other values—social, ethical, political—that are not usually seen as conducive to truth (from here on I'll just call these "values"). Values are understood to play a role in science in a number of straightforward ways: determining which research projects get pursued, motivating particular applications of scientific findings, and constraining the sorts of experiments scientists can do. So far, no problem: epistemic values play a role in scientific reasoning, and values play a role in guiding science. But do values themselves play a role in scientific reasoning?

The thesis known as the *value-free ideal* holds that values should not play a role in scientific reasoning itself, and if they do, that's a problem. For example, if a drug company publishes only studies that suggest their drug is effective and hides the results of studies that suggest their drug is ineffective, and goes on to make an inference based only on the publicly available evidence that their drug is effective, then the company is violating the value-free ideal. They would be engaged in a fancy form of wishful thinking. Many people hold that the value-free ideal is an important principle of science. However, there is a powerful challenge to the value-free ideal, and this challenge is especially worrying in applied sciences such as medical research.

The strongest argument against the value-free ideal is called the *argument from inductive risk*. Here it is. If we are deciding whether or not to accept or believe a hypothesis (H), there are two basic ways we could make a mistake: we could accept H when it is in fact false (call this a false positive) or we could reject H when it is in fact true (call this a false negative). These errors might have practical consequences: say, if H claims that chemical x causes cancer, and the production of x generates economic activity, then a false positive could harm such economic activity while a false negative could harm people's health.

The chances of committing these errors trade off against each other. For example, one way to completely avoid false positives would be to reject every hypothesis, in which case our false positive rate would be zero but our false negative rate would be high, and vice versa, one way to completely avoid false negatives would be to accept every hypothesis, in which case our false negative rate would be zero but our false positive rate would be high. And so on for intermediate cases. The research methods that are pertinent to H—including the characteriza-tion of data and modes of data analysis—can be tuned to minimize the chance of one type of error at the expense of increasing the chance of the other type of error. In so doing, the scientists who do that tuning import their values regarding the practical consequences of the two types of errors. Thus, the internal aspects of scientific reasoning are in-fluenced by values. Thus, the value-free ideal is impossible to satisfy, at least for hypotheses that pertain to practical contexts.

Some critics of the argument from inductive risk claim that a veiled premise of the argument is not compelling. The argument from induc-tive risk assumes that scientists must "accept" or "believe" a hypoth-esis. That is to assume that scientists must have an all-or-nothing epi-stemic attitude toward a hypothesis. But we will see in chapter 9 that a compelling epistemological model for scientific reasoning involves modeling beliefs as probabilities, in which epistemic attitudes toward hypotheses are not all-or-nothing, but rather are graded.

Another response to the argument from inductive risk is to reiter-ate that the value-free ideal is just that, an *ideal*, but like any ideal, just because the ability to satisfy the ideal in practice is limited does not tarnish the ideal itself. Consider the ideal of being perfectly hon-est. We know that not all people are perfectly honest. But this practi-cal shortcoming of the ideal does not mean that the ideal is false. It just means it is hard to achieve. As a rejoinder, one could note that the argument from inductive risk shows not just that the value-free ideal is hard to satisfy in practice, but that in certain domains it is, in principle, impossible to satisfy. If one holds the general view that ide-als that are in principle impossible to satisfy should not be guiding norms for us, then one will be more convinced by this defence of the argument from inductive risk. (Do you think that *ought* implies *can*? If so, you will be sympathetic to this challenge to the value-free ideal, and if not, then you won't.)

I have made much of the argument for inductive risk because it is an important challenge to an intuitive view that many hold about science, but also because it is especially applicable in medicine. Toxi-cology, for instance, has furnished articulations of the argument from inductive risk with compelling examples. The regulation of medical interventions also faces an argument from inductive risk: if regulators reject a new drug when it in fact is effective, then a valuable intervention is denied to patients and a company's financial interests are hurt, but if regulators approve a new drug when it in fact is ineffective or harmful, then resources are wasted, people are harmed, and other treatments are underutilized. Same with diagnosis: a false positive diagnosis carries the risk of overtreatment, while a false negative diagnosis carries the risk of undertreatment (see chapter 11). Each of these trade-offs opens the door for the influence of values. The considerations underlying the argument from inductive risk are important to many aspects of medicine.

If the value-free ideal is false, or at least impossible to satisfy in policy-oriented domains of science, this raises an important worry: *which* values should be permitted to influence the scientific process? Any values? Only select values? This is another type of demarcation problem.

Consider the hypothesis that claims that chemical x causes cancer. Suppose that x is produced in a factory, and there is a town two kilometers upriver from the town where many of the factory workers live, and there is another town ten kilometers downriver from the factory where few of the factory workers live. There is a worry that x is polluting the river, and there have been an unusual number of cases of cancer reported in the downstream town. In a case-control study, people with cancer were three times more likely to be living in the downstream town than the upstream town. In an experiment on rodents, large doses of x caused various sorts of tissue damage. For obvious ethical reasons scientists cannot do an RCT to test the effects of x.

Residents of the downstream town hire an epidemiologist, who argues that the case control study and the animal experiment indicate that x causes cancer, and though we cannot be certain, the health of people in the downstream town is at stake. The factory hires an epidemiologist, who argues that in the absence of an RCT, the case-control study and the animal experiment are inconclusive, and though we cannot be certain, the jobs of people in the upstream town are at stake, as is the financial well-being of the factory (along with the financial stake of the shareholders of the factory). So there are two competing social values at play: the value of people's health in the downstream town versus the value of people's jobs and other financial considerations in the upstream town. I suspect that many people have the intuition that the health of people in the downstream town should trump the employment and financial considerations of people in the upstream town. But what if the trade-off was a slightly higher rate of cancer in the downstream town versus the factory being forced to close, leading to widespread unemployment in the upstream town and shareholders in the factory losing a great deal of money? The challenge to the value-free ideal raises this unwelcome demarcation problem, namely, sorting out which values should be permitted to be taken into account when grappling with inductive risk, and how to balance competing values.

A related worry is this: Why should non-experts trust what experts say? If the inductive risk challenge to the value-free ideal is correct, then experts must rely in part on their values to proclaim matters of fact. But if a non-expert does not share the same values as the experts, then that non-expert can reason to a conclusion that differs from the expert's proclamation. Epistemic relativism threatens. Because the challenge to the value-free ideal gets off the ground in scientific contexts that have practical consequences—such as pharmaceutical regulation, toxicology, and climate science—this form of relativism is especially worrying.

A promising approach to salvage objectivity in the face of the above concerns—research biases, difficulties with demarcation principles, the inductive risk challenge to the value-free ideal—is to conceive of objectivity as arising out of features at the level of the scientific community. Perhaps the way that science is structurally organized can mitigate some of these threats to objectivity.

8.5 SOCIAL EPISTEMOLOGY

A reason science is admired is that many people hold it to be objective. But we have seen above that there is a variety of threats to such objectivity. Some philosophers hold that the best way to understand how science achieves objectivity, and concomitantly the most worrying threats to such objectivity, is to understand the social structure of science. Science is fundamentally a social enterprise, and the key to understanding its merits (and its drawbacks) is to elucidate the features that make it a social enterprise.

One of the most prominent theories of scientific objectivity that is based on the social nature of science is due to Helen Longino. According to Longino, individual scientists can be influenced by subjective, idiosyncratic biases, and their reasoning might be influenced by non-epistemic values, but the community of science has particular features that mitigate these subjective influences and can render science objective.

Start by considering the social nature of science. Individual scientists depend on each other for the conditions under which they practice—these conditions include the basic ideas they rely upon, the instruments they use, and the journals they publish in. Simply becoming a scientist involves a kind of initiation, requiring education and practical training, all of which is a social activity. Scientific activity is embedded in society—scientists receive funds from the public, and the ability to become a scientist requires basic public education. Ideally, both theories and evidence are publicly available and thus open to scrutiny.

The public nature of science affords criticism. Longino describes two important kinds of scientific criticism: evidential and conceptual. Evidential criticism challenges the extent to which a hypothesis is supported by evidence, challenges the internal and external validity of experiments, and challenges how such evidence is analyzed and reported. In the context of medical research, many of the features of methods noted in chapter 7 are foci for evidential criticism. Conceptual criticism challenges the soundness of hypotheses, challenges the consistency of particular hypotheses with more general and better-accepted theories, and challenges the relevance of particular pieces of evidence for a hypothesis. In the context of medical research, such criticism could invoke some of the issues regarding theories of disease, causal models of disease, and nosology noted in chapters 2 through 5.

Objectivity is achieved if these kinds of criticism can expose the influence of subjective biases in research and ideally block such influence. For example, in 1998 a physician, Andrew Wakefield, published a very controversial article in the prestigious medical journal *The Lancet* that suggested that the MMR vaccine (measles, mumps, and rubella) could cause autism. This influenced some parents to not vaccinate their children, which in turn led to increased rates of measles infections. Critics noted many problems with the research behind this article—including the manipulation of evidence and the fact that the author of the article had undeclared conflicts of interest—and so the journal subsequently retracted the article.

Such criticism can also lead to scientific innovations in an attempt to respond to criticisms. A slightly older example from medicine provides a good illustration of a case in which the target of criticism ultimately survived thanks to scientific innovation. The first studies suggesting that smoking causes lung cancer were published in the 1950s, led by the epidemiologist Sir Bradford Hill. The problem was that these were case-control studies. (Can you remember from chapter 7 what the major shortcoming of case-control studies is?) This study compared the smoking rates between those people diagnosed with lung cancer against a set of control subjects who had not been diagnosed with lung cancer, and found a much higher smoking rate among those with lung cancer. The question was this: Does smoking *cause* lung cancer? The eminent statistician Ronald Fisher argued that Hill's finding could be due to a confounding factor, or what philosophers call a "common cause"—perhaps there is a gene that both increases the chances that a person will smoke and increases the chances that a person will get lung cancer.

If Fisher was correct, then the correlation between smoking and lung cancer would not indicate that smoking causes lung cancer. Hill responded by arguing that one can justify causal inferences by appealing to a variety of kinds of evidence, including mechanistic evidence, dose-response relations, and evidence from case-control studies. This became known as the "Hill criteria," which are really more like a set of reasonable, albeit vague, guidelines on how to justify causal inferences in epidemiology. The Hill criteria have been very influential in epidemiological research, and resulted in part from Fisher's criticisms (see §9.2).

Let's return to Longino's theory of objectivity. We have seen the importance that Longino places on the role of criticism for science to achieve objectivity. However, other domains of life involve public criticism, such as art, politics, and religion. Thus, criticism alone is insufficient for an activity to achieve objectivity. But science has another distinctive feature: it is empirical. Scientific activity is based on observations and experiments. Longino's theory is that the combination of empiricism plus criticism allows science to achieve objectivity. And both the empirical and the critical nature of science are social.

In order for this recipe for objectivity to work, Longino claims that criticism should be transformative. That is, scientific criticism should lead to changes in scientific methods, assumptions, and conclusions. For criticism to be transformative there are a few features that a scientific community must have: there must be recognized avenues for criticism, such as journals and grant applications; there must be shared standards within the scientific community; the community must be responsive to criticism; and there must be some degree of shared intellectual authority. Each of these criteria requires scientific disciplines to be structured as a community with particular norms. Journals and peer review, for example, help to keep non-mainstream views out; having shared standards also involves a gate-keeping function such that whimsical outsiders' criticisms do not have much influence; in order for intellectual authority to be roughly shared, some scientists have to become and be recognized as experts. The sharing of intellectual authority also helps diverse perspectives participate in scientific criticism, and this diversity of perspectives itself aids in achieving objectivity.

This way of thinking about scientific objectivity faces its own demarcation problems. Longino notes that criticism can't go on forever—especially in practical scientific contexts like medicine, sometimes criticism must be curtailed because decisions must be made. Moreover, the structuring of a scientific community involves distinguishing some people as experts and some as non-experts: the former get shared intellectual authority and the privilege of articulating criticism that is responded to, while the latter do not. Here are the demarcation problems for this social view of objectivity: *Which* criticisms should be responded to? *Who* counts as an expert endowed with intellectual authority? To what *degree* should a community be responsive to criticism?

Think back to the MMR vaccine controversy. In one sense the medical community was responsive to Wakefield's article, in that many medical scientists denounced it. But in another sense—in the sense of actual vaccine practices—medicine did not budge, and nor should it have. Another question that arises in thinking about knowledge at a social level is this: What is the significance of disagreement among experts? Longino's theory holds that objectivity is achieved through active criticism among members of a scientific community. But what if that community cannot agree on an important scientific question? Does the community need to come to consensus on the subject? Or something less than consensus?

Medical research implements some aspects of social epistemology, as exemplified by Longino's theory. There are recognized avenues for criticism, and there are shared standards. An example of a widely shared standard is the regulatory standard for the approval of a new drug—the approval standard in several jurisdictions, including the FDA, is that there must be two "positive" RCTs that suggest a new drug is better than placebo (discussed in chapter 14), where "positive" means statistically significant according to frequentist statistics (to recall problems with this standard discussed in chapter 7, think of the example of the trial on retroactive intercessory prayer; we'll see additional problems with the standard in chapter 9). For an example of attempting to facilitate experts' critical engagements with each other and to develop consensus, consider the practice of medical scientists and policy-makers to sometimes convene "consensus conferences." These are meetings designed to publicly collect and criticize evidence and hypotheses (as noted above, there is some debate among philosophers about just how important consensus is, and in this context there is some debate about how effective consensus conferences can be at actually achieving consensus).

Medical science does not always live up to the norms of theories like Longino's—other aspects of medical research violate features of this social theory of objectivity. For example, publication bias is a practice in which the ideal of sharing evidence publicly is thwarted.

A virtue of Longino's theory of objectivity is that it can tell us what is wrong with a practice such as publication bias—because it keeps evidence out of public view, it minimizes the possibility of criticism, and since criticism is a crucial ingredient for achieving objectivity, such a practice threatens objectivity.

FURTHER READING

Theories of objectivity: Douglas (2004)

Publication bias: Biddle (2007)

Inductive risk: Douglas (2000), Wilholt (2009), Elliott (2011), John (2011), Brown (2013)

Social epistemology: Longino (1990), Solomon (2001), Miller (2013), de Melo-Martin and Intemann (2011), Jukola (2015)

Consensus and dissent: Solomon (2011), Miller (2013), Biddle (2013), Solomon (2015)

Conflicts of interest: Krimsky (2003), Resnik (2007), Ioannidis (2011), Pinto (2015)

DISCUSSION QUESTIONS

1. Medical science occurs in a social context. Is this social context a problem for the objectivity of science? Explain.
2. The argument from inductive risk purports to show that non-epistemic values influence the internal workings of scientific reasoning. Is this a threat to scientific objectivity? Explain.
3. Some people argue that a diversity of perspectives should be included in the planning, performance, and analysis of medical science. Why? Why can't medical science just be purely "evidence-based"? What good, if any, is gained by the incorporation of these various perspectives?
4. What role should non-epistemic values play in biomedical research?

9 : INFERENCE

Some of the numerous challenges facing scientists who test the effectiveness of medical interventions were the subject of §7.3. In addition to those methodological challenges, there is another, and arguably more fundamental, kind of challenge pertinent to medical research: the choice of an inductive framework or theory of inference. In short, once we have evidence, we must make inferences on the basis of that evidence. How should we do that? There are several related issues packed into this question.

The first issue is this: What sort of evidence should our inferences about medical interventions be based on? We have already seen, in chapter 7, some views that pertain directly or indirectly to this question. Proponents of evidence-based medicine, and many regulatory agencies, are committed to the view that we only need to use evidence from randomized trials about a medical intervention to make an inference about the effectiveness of that intervention. We also saw that the mechanista position denies this and holds instead that we ought to inform such inferences by appealing to knowledge of relevant mechanisms.

The second issue is this: How should that evidence be used? What form should such inferences take? Again, the dominant view among regulators and evidence-based medicine is that evidence from randomized trials can be used directly, to make a very simple inference about the effectiveness of an intervention. In this chapter we will see criticisms of this view. The critical view argues that inferences about effectiveness cannot be direct, but rather must be modulated in various ways. This chapter examines the various ways that causal inference goes beyond direct inference from randomized trials. Moreover, before data from studies can be used in a causal inference, the data have to be quantitatively summarized in particular ways, but there are multiple possible ways to do this, and these can lead to different judgments about effectiveness.

The third issue is this: How should statistics inform our inference? Causal inference in medicine is almost always statistical in nature. The two main theories of scientific inference are frequentism and Bayesianism, and each has merits and drawbacks. We will assess these two theories of statistical inference here.

This chapter is perhaps the most technical of the book. But it is important to learn this technicalia because much recent philosophy of science and medicine uses these technical tools, and these tools help us to properly understand medicine.

9.2 CAUSAL INFERENCE

The main type of question that medical scientists want to answer is causal in nature. Will this drug lower my blood pressure? Does smoking cause lung cancer? Do antidepressants cause harmful side effects? What kind of bacterium causes this infection?

We saw in chapter 7 that one position about causal inference in medicine is that randomized trials are both necessary and sufficient for causal inference. We called this the black box thesis. The idea is that if a randomized trial, or a meta-analysis of randomized trials, provides evidence that d causes x, then we are justified in inferring that d causes x. The mechanista thesis is opposed to the black box thesis for a number of reasons. The main criticism of the black box thesis amounted to arguing that evidence that d causes x from a randomized trial is insufficient to infer that d causes x. Another concern is that for many causal inferences we want to make, we simply do not have access to randomized trials. This is especially the case for toxicological hypotheses, such as "this industrial chemical causes cancer," because we cannot ethically perform a randomized trial in which we give some subjects a substance that we have reason to think causes harm. If randomized trials are necessary for causal inference, then we could never have grounds to make such inferences (this might be convenient for the manufacturers of toxicological substances but inconvenient for those who are hurt by them).

We saw earlier a famous episode that illustrates this. In the mid-twentieth century, case-control studies suggested that there was a link between smoking and lung cancer. The question was: does smoking *cause* lung cancer? The statistician Fisher claimed that the correlation between smoking and lung cancer that was observed in these case-control studies could be due to an unknown common cause of both smoking and lung cancer. Perhaps, suggested Fisher, there is a genetic factor that increases the probability that one smokes and also increases the probability that one will get lung cancer. If so, then the case-control studies did not provide evidence that smoking causes lung cancer. Fisher's implication was that a randomized trial would be necessary to show that smoking causes lung cancer. In response, the epidemiologist Hill argued that these studies, together with other considerations, did provide grounds for causal inference.

Hill enumerated the other considerations that he claimed could, when taken together, provide grounds for causal inference even in the absence of evidence from randomized trials. These considerations have become known as "Hill's criteria" (though they are not, strictly speaking, criteria, but are better thought of as heuristics for causal inference). The Hill criteria are as follows:

1. Strength of association: a strong association between possible cause and possible effect is more likely to be genuinely causal than a weak association.
2. Consistency of results: an association between possible cause and possible effect that is observed in multiple studies is more likely to be genuinely causal.
3. Specificity: a specific cause has a specific effect; correlations between coarse-grained or non-specific possible causes and effects provide less evidence for a true causal relation than correlations between specific possible causes and effects.
4. Temporality: a cause precedes its effect.
5. Biological gradient: a dose-response pattern of association between possible cause and effect is evidence of a true causal relation.
6. Plausibility: a plausible biological mechanism that can explain a correlation is evidence of a true causal relation.
7. Coherence: a causal interpretation of an association should cohere with other established knowledge.

8. Experimental evidence: when available, evidence from controlled experiments should be considered.
9. Analogy: analogies with other known causal relations can aid in causal inference; if the possible causal relation is similar to a known causal relation, then there is some reason to think that the possible causal relation is real.

These considerations, argued Hill, can together provide a strong inductive basis for causal inference. Notice that some of these considerations are basically those that mechanistas in §7.7 argued are important for causal inference (especially considerations 6, 7, and 9). The important point that Hill wanted to establish is that even in the absence of evidence from randomized trials, these considerations can serve as evidence to warrant causal inferences.

Another well-known set of criteria used to establish causation is known as "Koch's postulates," named after the physician and microbiologist Robert Koch. At the end of the nineteenth century Koch wanted to establish the physical basis for particular infectious diseases. The germ theory of disease had recently been established, and Koch's postulates were criteria meant to help researchers identify the microorganism that is responsible for a particular disease. His postulates are as follows:

1. The organism must be found in all individuals who have the disease but should not be found in disease-free individuals.
2. The organism must be isolated from a diseased individual and grown in culture.
3. The cultured organism should cause disease when introduced into a healthy individual.
4. The organism must be isolated from the newly inoculated individual and identified as the same kind of organism that caused the original disease.

Of course, we now know that there are asymptomatic individuals who have organisms that can cause infectious diseases, so (1) is too strong. Also, some infectious agents, such as viruses, cannot be grown in pure culture, and so (2) must be relaxed. In any case, Koch's postulates are clearly intended for guiding inferences regarding what kind of organism is responsible for a particular infectious disease, and thus the set of criteria is not a general theory of causal inference for medical science.

Can there be a general theory of causal inference for medicine? Perhaps. But we should take care to note that there are a variety of kinds of causal inferences that are important in medicine. In chapter 11 we examine diagnosis, which is often thought to be an explanatory causal inference. This chapter is concerned with causal inferences about the effectiveness of medical interventions, which are, in a clinical context, predictive causal inferences. The fundamental question is this: How ought we measure the effectiveness of medical interventions?

9.3 EXTRAPOLATION

We investigated extrapolation in the context of animal models in chapter 7. Another important issue about extrapolation arises in the context of human research. Extrapolation is a kind of causal inference. The key question addressed in this section is this: If we find that d causes x in a base human population, under what conditions can we infer that d causes x in a target population? A concern about extrapolation is especially pressing when the population from which the evidence was generated (the "base" population) is likely to be different from the population for which we want to make the causal inference (the "target" population).

As we saw earlier, evidence-based medicine holds that the best form of evidence comes from randomized trials. A randomized trial involves selecting subjects in a very particular way—trials employ "inclusion criteria" and "exclusion criteria" to determine the kinds of people that are included as subjects. Then the subjects are randomized to the intervention group and control group, and the administration of both the intervention and the control (placebo or competitor intervention) is done in a careful manner, constrained by instructions stipulated by the planners of the trial. Thus, many features of the trial context, especially the features of the subject population and the administration of the interventions, differ from features in the wild (the target population in the real world clinical context). Obviously we hope that evidence from the trial can be used to make predictions about what will happen when physicians use the tested intervention in the wild. But how? To use the terminology from chapter 7, can we reliably use simple extrapolation? Or do we need a more sophisticated theory of extrapolation, like the mechanism-based extrapolation we studied for animal models?

In evidence-based medicine the working assumption is that when it comes to extrapolating from trials to the wild, simple extrapolation is fine. For instance, according to some of the leading medical scientists in evidence-based medicine, in order to determine whether one can extrapolate the results from clinical trials to a particular patient, one should "ask whether there is some compelling reason why the results should not be applied to the patient. A compelling reason usually won't be found, and most often you can generalise the results to your patient with confidence" (Guyatt and Rennie 2001). This is a little more sophisticated than simple extrapolation, since the claim is that one should determine whether there are reasons why simple extrapolation is unjustified. Nevertheless, the guidance claims that such reasons are rare, and that simple extrapolation should be the default assumption.

Critics of this argue that in typical cases simple extrapolation should not be the default assumption, because there are usually reasons to expect that results in a base population will not hold in the target population. Some of these differences were noted above: features of patients in the wild will very likely differ from features of the carefully selected subjects in a trial. Also, a patient in the wild will tend to have a very different experience in their clinical setting than subjects in trials. A defender of simple extrapolation could respond by claiming that these are differences that usually don't make a difference—that is, this response holds that the different features of patients in the wild and their experience in the clinical setting, compared with subjects in trials, should not make a difference to whether or not a drug is effective. However, many of these differences have been shown to influence the effectiveness of interventions in empirical studies. For example, a patient's age, gender, severity of illness, and number of pre-existing medications all influence the effectiveness of a medical intervention, and these are the features that often determine whether or not a person can be a subject in a trial.

Another problem with simple extrapolation is that if we base our predictions about patients in the wild on the results of published randomized trials, our predictions often will be based on an incomplete body of evidence, due to publication bias (see chapter 8). Publication bias usually results in artificial inflations of estimates of effectiveness, and so simple extrapolation based on published evidence inherits this tendency to overestimate effectiveness.

Finally, an issue that arose in the context of extrapolating from animals to humans may be pertinent in the context of extrapolating from one human population to another: simple extrapolation ignores details about the mechanism undergirding a causal relation. If a trial produces evidence that d causes x, but our background knowledge about the mechanisms relevant to d and x make it unlikely that d could cause x, then using simple extrapolation to predict that d will cause x in a target population would be unwise. A good illustration of this problem is the trial suggesting that retroactive intercessory prayer can improve patients' health (discussed in chapter 7). Surely we should not extrapolate from this finding, and since simple extrapolation says we should, that suggests that there is a problem with simple extrapolation.

We learned briefly about the difference between case-control studies and randomized trials (§7.2). In §9.2 we saw that the Hill criteria were meant to apply to scenarios in which we do not have access to randomized trials but do have access to other kinds of evidence. Case-control studies can be more reliable when it comes to extrapolation than randomized trials because case-control studies are usually done on subjects in the wild. Like randomized trials, usually case-control studies have criteria for selecting which subjects to gather data on, but those criteria are far looser than subject selection criteria for randomized trials, and so subjects in case-control studies are more like the target population than subjects in randomized trials. (That said, case-control studies are much more likely to suffer from other forms of bias, as we learned earlier.) Hill's criteria can be taken as a general strategy for extrapolation. The idea is that if we want to make an inference about whether or not d causes x in a target population, we ought to take into account as much evidence as we can, including the various kinds of evidence referred to by Hill's criteria.

9.4 MEASURING EFFECTIVENESS

Let's finally face the question head on. Once we have data from a randomized trial about a medical intervention, how should we use that data to make a causal inference about the effectiveness of that intervention?

We've already seen that there are several aspects to this question. One is about what evidence should be appealed to in the first place—the question presupposes that evidence from trials must be appealed to. The debate we saw in several earlier sections was about whether or not other forms of evidence should be relied on. Another aspect to the question about inferring effectiveness is about extrapolation. An inference about effectiveness involves extrapolation, and some people think that extrapolation involves a direct inference from evidence gathered from a trial (or base) population to claims about a target population, while others think that extrapolation is more nuanced than this, and, again, relies on more kinds of evidence than merely data from randomized trials.

There is another, more technical, issue. Data from trials must be summarized in various ways to render it into evidence for a causal hypothesis. These summaries are called "outcome measures" or "effect sizes." An outcome measure is a formal description of the relation between the value of a measured property in one group of a trial and the value of that property in the other group of the trial. For example, suppose a trial measures levels of depression in a group that is given a drug and in a group that gets a placebo; an outcome measure compares the values of those depression levels between the two groups. When actual data is available and plugged into an outcome measure, you get an "effect size." There are many outcome measures available for medical scientists. It turns out that one's choice of outcome measures can influence one's causal inferences.

TABLE 1. *Two-by-two table for defining outcome measures*

Group	Outcome	
	Y	N
E	a	b
C	c	d

It's easiest to see this by considering outcome measures for binary features (like "dead or alive"). The most common binary outcome measures are relative risk (sometimes called risk ratio), relative risk reduction, risk difference (sometimes called absolute risk reduction), and number needed to treat. To understand what these are, we refer to a "two-by-two table" (Table 1). This table is constructed by imagining a trial that has a group that receives the experimental intervention (E), and a group that receives a control (C) (which could be a placebo or a competitor intervention). At the end of the trial a binary outcome is either present (Y) or absent (N). The number of subjects with these outcomes in the two groups is given by letters a, b, c, and d, as indicated in the table.

The most common outcome measures are defined by reference to the two-by-two table.

Relative risk (RR) is defined as:

$$RR = [a/(a+b)] / [c/(c+d)]$$

Relative risk reduction (RRR) is defined as:

$$RRR = [[a/(a+b)]-[c/(c+d)]] / [c/(c+d)]$$

Risk difference (RD) is defined as:

$$RD = a/(a+b)-c/(c+d)$$

Number needed to treat (NNT) is defined as:

$$NNT = 1 / |[a/(a+b)]-[c/(c+d)]|$$

There are a few details about these outcome measures that are worth describing, which make them easier to understand. RR is the proportion of subjects in the experimental group with a Y outcome, divided

TABLE 2. *Two-by-two table for a hypothetical trial*

Group	Outcome	
	Dead	Alive
Drug	6	94
Placebo	8	92

by the proportion of subjects in the control group with a Y outcome. In contrast, RD is the difference between these proportions. Finally, NNT is just the inverse of RD—so if the RD is 4%, or 0.04, NNT would be 1/0.04, which is 25.

Let's consider an example. Table 2 is a two-by-two table from a hypothetical trial testing the capacity of a drug to lower the risk of death.

$$\text{RR} = [6/(6+94)] / [8/(8+92)]$$
$$= 0.06/0.08$$
$$= 0.75$$
$$\text{RRR} = [[6/(6+94)]-[8/(8+92)]] / [8/(8+92)]$$
$$= -0.25$$
$$= -25\%$$
$$\text{RD} = [6/(6+94)]-[8/(8+92)]$$
$$= -0.02$$
$$= -2\%$$
$$\text{NNT} = 1 / |-0.02|$$
$$= 50$$

Now, in words. The relative risk of dying when on the drug is 0.75 compared to when on placebo. The relative risk reduction is 25%; one way to say that is the risk of dying is 25% lower in the drug group compared with the placebo group. The risk difference, on the other hand, is only 2%, so taking the drug lowers an individual's risk of death by 2%. Finally, the number needed to treat is 50, so we would have to give 50 people the drug in order to avoid one death (and thus, 49 people would take the drug without that benefit).

Suppose we are interested in estimating the effectiveness of the drug at lowering the risk of death. From this one study, we have a few effect sizes that we could use as the basis of our inference. Should we use the relative risk reduction, in which case the inference would begin by noting that the drug appears to lower the risk of death by 25%? Or should we use the risk difference, in which case the inference would begin by noting that the drug appears to decrease the probability of dying by 2%?

Most published articles reporting the results of trials state the relative risk or relative risk reduction, but not the risk difference. Some critics have noted that these relative measures are very misleading. Here's their argument. Relative risk reduction tells you the proportion—among the people who would have had the bad outcome (in this case, death)—of people who avoid that bad outcome with the intervention. The problem is that real patients don't know if they would be among those people who would have had the bad outcome. If the outcome is rare, like death in a given period of time, then chances are low that a person would have the outcome. What people need in order to make an informed treatment decision, argue these critics, is the proportion of people who avoid the bad outcome with the intervention, compared to placebo, among *all* people in the trial, and not just the people who would have had the bad outcome. The outcome measure that represents this crucial information is the risk difference.

Notice that in this example the risk difference appears much smaller than the relative risk reduction. This is generally the case when the outcome in question is rare. This fact is important. Psychological research shows that people are bad at reasoning with probabilities (in the next section we learn a little about probability theory). Some studies suggest that we have a tendency to confuse probabilities like the relative risk reduction with probabilities like the risk difference. This can lead to gross overestimates of the effectiveness of medical interventions. This could explain why other studies show that physicians are more willing to prescribe interventions, and patients are more willing to consume those interventions, when presented with relative outcome measures compared with the risk difference, and physicians and patients more accurately estimate effectiveness when presented with risk difference.

There is still another nuance to measuring the effectiveness of medical interventions. Based on some of the things we learned in chapters 7 and 8, we know that medical research typically has various forms of bias. The "direct inference" view held by evidence-based medicine and regulators involves simply making an inference about the effectiveness of medical interventions on the basis of effect sizes from trials, but this amounts to neglecting the influence of these known biases. Somehow we ought to modulate our inferences by taking into account what we know about the context of medical research. It's not obvious how best to do this. One possibility is to *model* effectiveness, roughly in the same way that climate modelers make predictions about future climate states based on models, or the way that physicists predict the dynamic motion of projectile objects on the basis of the various forces that influence such motion—the idea is, when making an effectiveness inference, we ought to incorporate factors that represent the various biases in medical research, a bit like the incorporation of friction when predicting the motion of objects. Another possibility is to model the measurement of effectiveness in epistemic terms. This is an approach that can be aided with the use of probabilities, which is the subject of the next section.

9.5 THEORIES OF STATISTICAL INFERENCE

There are two competing theories of statistical inference: frequentism and Bayesianism. Both theories are used in medical research—for most of the twentieth century frequentism was the favored approach, but now Bayesianism is gaining popularity. The two theories differ on some fundamental issues and can reach differing conclusions for particular inferences. Despite the popularity of frequentism among practicing scientists, Bayesianism is favored by most philosophers and is now becoming more prominent among epidemiologists and other medical scientists.

Before diving into the technical details of these two theories of statistical inference, let's start with a story about a mind-reading salmon. Researchers presented a salmon with pictures of people showing emotions, and scanned the salmon's brain using fMRI. They found that when the salmon saw pictures of people with emotions, regions of its brains were stimulated—and this finding was statistically significant (it had a very low "p-value," which, as we'll see below, is said to be a good thing by many researchers). As if this were not surprising enough, it turns out that the salmon was dead. What can we learn from the fact that this finding was statistically significant? Should we conclude that the dead salmon was able to infer the emotional states of the people it saw in photographs?

Okay, now let's learn about the two theories of statistical inference. If you are puzzled about what to make of the dead mind-reading salmon, hopefully this brief foray into the foundations of the two leading schools of statistics will help.

Bayesians maintain that our beliefs can be modeled as probabilities. (It's named after Thomas Bayes, a British statistician and philosopher in the eighteenth century.) If you completely disbelieve a hypothesis, this means you assign a probability of 0 to the hypothesis; if you are certain of the hypothesis, this means you assign a probability of 1 to it; and if you're sitting on the fence about the hypothesis, this means you might assign a probability of around 0.5 to it. An important idea for Bayesianism is called a "conditional probability." This tool is used by philosophers of science for many purposes, including modeling scientific reasoning and defining important scientific concepts such as causation and explanation, and it can also help in practical contexts in medicine such as screening and diagnosis (see chapter 11).

A conditional probability takes the form of a statement "the probability of A, given B"—the probability that it is raining outside, given that I'm in England, for example. To express conditional probabilities we write $P(A|B)$ to represent "the probability of A given B." Probabilities must satisfy certain axioms, and there is a powerful theorem, called Bayes' Theorem, that allows one to unpack conditional probabilities in useful ways. Here it is:

$$P(A|B) = P(B|A)P(A) / P(B)$$

One can find easy proofs of Bayes' Theorem in probability textbooks or online. The theorem is relevant to scientific inference because we can represent inference about a hypothesis (H), upon receiving evidence (E), as a conditional probability: P(H|E). So scientific inference can be modeled according to Bayes' Theorem:

$$P(H|E) = P(E|H)P(H)/P(E)$$

The term on the left side of the equation is called the "posterior probability," and it represents your final confidence in the hypothesis once you've received the evidence. The first term on the right side of the equation, P(E|H), is called the "likelihood," and it represents the fit between the hypothesis and the evidence—another way some people think about the likelihood is that it measures the extent to which H explains E. The next term, P(H), is called the "prior probability of the hypothesis," and it represents your prior confidence in the hypothesis before seeing the new evidence. The final term, P(E), is called the "prior probability of the evidence" (or the "expectancy" of the evidence), and it represents how surprising or compelling the evidence is.

Before proceeding we must note a more detailed version of Bayes' Theorem. The term P(E) can be expanded to give this version of the theorem:

$$P(H|E) = P(E|H)P(H) / [P(E|H)P(H) + P(E|{\sim}H)P({\sim}H)]$$

Here ~H represents "not H," so P(~H) means "the probability that H is false."

Note how intuitive it is to model our confidence or belief in hypotheses using probabilities. If it is autumn in Vancouver, how confident are you that it is going to rain? Perhaps somewhere around 60% confident? So your probability in the hypothesis "it is going to rain" would be 0.6. If your hypothesis (H) is "it will rain today" then your P(H) would be 0.6. Suppose now you look out the window and see dark clouds. Your evidence (E) is "there are dark clouds outside." This might change your confidence in it raining today to 80%; that is, P(H|E) would be 0.8. There are technical arguments that show that it is irrational to not follow Bayes' Theorem when making inferences. We won't study those arguments here, but I hope you will agree that modeling scientific inference using probabilities makes sense.

The other main school of scientific inference is called *frequentism*. This statistical approach is much more common in medical science. The main tool of inference for frequentism is called a *significance test*. This involves stating a "null hypothesis" for an experiment, which in the context of medical research is usually a hypothesis that the intervention is ineffective. If H is a hypothesis that the intervention is effective, then ~H represents that H is false: ~H is the null hypothesis (or, in other words, the hypothesis that the intervention makes no difference to the measured outcomes). After the data (E) from the study has been gathered, a "p-value" is calculated, which is the probability that we would get the data that we in fact got if the null hypothesis were true: $P(E|\sim H)$. Frequentist statisticians hold that if the p-value is very low, say, 0.01 or 0.05, then the null hypothesis should be rejected. The next (controversial) step is to infer H. Many frequentists warn again this last step, but in practice it is widespread (see §13.4 on standards for regulation, for example).

Critics argue that both the "reject ~H" step and the "infer H" step of frequentist inferences are invalid. Let's first consider the "reject ~H" step. The inference rule of the "reject ~H" step is: if $P(E|\sim H)$ is low, reject ~H. But this is not generally valid. Here is a counter-example. Suppose I have two jars each containing marbles of various colors. Jar 1 has 97% red marbles and Jar 2 has 99.9% red marbles. I hand you one of the jars, but you don't know which one it is. You reach into the jar and randomly pull out a blue marble. That is your evidence (E). Suppose your null hypothesis (~H) is that you have Jar 1. Note that $P(E|\sim H)$ is very low. But rejecting ~H would be fallacious, because your evidence confirms ~H more than it disconfirms ~H. The blue marble supports the hypothesis that you have Jar 1 much more than it supports the hypothesis that you have Jar 2. Even though your p-value for the null hypothesis is low, it would be unwise to reject the null hypothesis.

Consider next the inference rule of the "accept H" step of frequentist inferences. To accept H once we have our evidence E, we should demand that the posterior probability, $P(H|E)$, is quite high. But recall the full version of Bayes' Theorem above. To infer $P(H|E)$, we need a lot more than the p-value, which merely gives us $P(E|\sim H)$.

If $P(E|\sim H)$ is very low, that is a long way from being able to conclude that $P(H|E)$ is high. Perhaps most importantly, what is ignored in this step is $P(H)$, the prior probability of H. The prior probability is informed by one's background beliefs, previously gathered evidence, and other theories. Inferences that ignore the prior probability commit what is called the "base-rate fallacy" (because prior probabilities are also referred to as base rates). To reiterate, a scientific inference is concerned with determining $P(H|E)$, and, as can be seen in Bayes' Theorem, this is directly proportional to $P(H)$.

Consider again the trial that tested retroactive intercessory prayer. Before seeing any evidence from this trial, what would be your prior probability that retroactive intercessory prayer is effective? To think that this intervention could be effective you would have to hold beliefs that are inconsistent with fundamental laws of physics: for instance, you would have to think that one's actions could influence events in the past. Thus the prior probability that this intervention is effective ought to be extremely low, and no matter what evidence is reported in the trial, no matter how low the p-values are, because the posterior probability that the intervention is effective should be influenced by the prior probability, the posterior probability also ought to be low. To take another example, recall the dead mind-reading salmon from above: to "accept H" would amount to believing that this dead salmon's brain was activated in various ways upon seeing photographs of human emotions. But that is extremely implausible. In short, the "accept H" step in the frequentist inference is fallacious because it ignores a great deal of information that is relevant to the plausibility of H.

This is a long-winded way of saying that it was reasonable for you to not believe in the effectiveness of retroactive intercessory prayer even after I told you about the evidence from the trial that tested it, because that is exactly what Bayesianism would recommend. Note, too, the similarity between the discussion about the prior probability of the hypothesis and the discussion in the previous section about the mechanista thesis. If we want to make an inference about the probability that an intervention is effective, one way of understanding the importance of taking into account the prior probability that the intervention is effective is that we ought to take into account knowledge about how the intervention works mechanistically or pathophysiologically. The retroactive intercessory prayer example shows that, in some cases at least, failing to take into account mechanistic evidence as the black box thesis urges amounts to committing the base-rate fallacy.

To summarize the above critical remarks regarding frequentism, a fundamental problem with this theory of statistical inference is that it will lead to many false positive findings (it also leads to false negative findings—the argument for this is pretty straightforward and I leave it to you as an exercise).

The above remarks make it seem as if Bayesianism is clearly superior to frequentism. But Bayesianism also has its problems. Perhaps the biggest problem involves determining the value of P(H). Critics of Bayesianism say that in real scientific cases there is no objective way to determine the value of this term, and instead Bayesians must rely on subjective assessments of the prior probability of the hypothesis. This subjectivity is said to be a damning criticism of a theory of scientific inference, which one might think ought to be objective. To this, Bayesians reply that this subjectivity is a faithful representation of the nature of science, which often relies on expertise and judgment and other subjective elements. Determining P(H) isn't totally unconstrained, say Bayesians—scientists still have to appeal to reasons and evidence—but ultimately there is a role for subjective judgment in the Bayesian theory of inference. Indeed, Bayesians claim that it is a virtue of their theory of inference that it explicitly articulates the role of subjective judgment in scientific inference, rather than pretend that there is no subjectivity in science.

9.6 TESTING PRECISION MEDICINE

Some argue that the regulatory standards that stipulate how medical interventions must be tested are cumbersome and should, in some cases at least, be lowered. Precision medicine makes this problem acute. Recall that precision medicine involves the articulation of more fine-grained disease categories. It follows that fewer people will be diagnosed with a particular disease. If a medical intervention is in fact precise, in that it targets only the physiological basis of a fine-grained disease category, then that intervention will help fewer people. It will be harder to perform large phase 3 trials on such interventions because there will be fewer subjects available for trials.

To address this problem, one approach is to require only the smaller phase 2 trials in testing precision interventions. If the intervention is in fact precise, then we should expect it to be very effective, and this effectiveness will show up in a smaller trial. Indeed, the only reason we need large trials is that they are necessary to demonstrate small effects of interventions. Statisticians call the "power" of a trial the ability of a trial to detect a certain effect size of an intervention. Trial power is directly proportional to both an intervention's effect size and the number of people in the trial. All else being equal, as the effect size of an intervention goes up, so does the power of the trial, and hence the trial needs fewer subjects with larger effect sizes to achieve equivalent power. Since the presupposition of precision medicine is that precise interventions will be very effective and hence have large effect sizes, it follows that trials testing precision interventions would require fewer subjects to achieve satisfactory power. Thus we can revise regulatory standards on the basis of the promise of precision medicine—let's call this the optimistic view of precision medicine, which holds a corresponding revisionist view of how precision medicines must be tested.

One worry about lowering epistemic standards for regulation is that regulatory standards can already be manipulated for industrial profit. Given the powerful financial incentives in medicine that can motivate biased research, we should be raising epistemic standards rather than lowering them. Another worry is that a premise of the above argument is that the lowered standards ought to apply only when the medical intervention in question is "precise" (chapter 4). Knowing that an intervention operates precisely requires having a good understanding of the pathophysiological basis of the disease in question and having a good understanding of the mechanism by which the intervention operates on this pathophysiology. Sometimes we have such knowledge. But the pathophysiological basis of many diseases is extremely complex, and the mechanism of action of many interventions is also extremely complex, so in many cases we could be duped into thinking that we have a good understanding of the precise nature of interventions when in fact we do not. Finally, there have been very few good examples of precision medicine actually succeeding at what it aims to do. For these reasons, regulatory standards should not be lowered for precision medicine—let's call this the pessimistic view of precision medicine, which holds a corresponding conservative view of how precision medicines must be tested.

Should we be optimists or pessimists about precision medicine? Should we be revisionists or conservatives when it comes to regulatory standards for how precision medicines should be tested?

FURTHER READING

Theories of statistical inference: Mayo (1996), Howson and Urbach (1989), Sober (2008), Sprenger (2014)
Measuring effectiveness: McClimans (2013), Stegenga (2015a)
Testing precision medicine: Teira (2017)
Extrapolation: Tonelli (2006), Steel (2007), Fuller and Flores (2015)

DISCUSSION QUESTIONS

1. Are RCTs necessary and/or sufficient for making inferences about the effectiveness of medical interventions?
2. Are the epistemological principles of evidence-based medicine convincing? Begin by articulating what evidence-based medicine is, and then evaluate one or more of its principles.
3. Describe how mechanistic evidence is supposed to ground causal inference. Then, find a case study and explain whether, in that instance, knowledge of mechanisms was necessary or at least useful to infer causation.
4. What are the two main theories of statistical inference? Which one is better? Why?

10 : EFFECTIVENESS, SKEPTICISM, AND ALTERNATIVES

10.1 SUMMARY

What does it mean to call a medical intervention effective? In one obvious sense, to say that a medical intervention is effective is just to say that the intervention has the capacity to improve health. But this can't be all there is to effectiveness, because many things improve health yet are not typically deemed medical interventions (let alone *effective* medical interventions): exercise, nutritious diet, and meditation are a few examples. This chapter starts by examining various positions on what is required for a medical intervention to be deemed effective.

With that in hand, we can address a long-standing debate among physicians, epidemiologists, and philosophers: is medicine effective? Surprisingly, many healthcare practitioners and medical scientists (and a few philosophers) have raised doubts about the capacity of medicine to generally and significantly improve health by targeting diseases. This skeptical view is sometimes called *therapeutic nihilism* or *medical nihilism*. We will assess the arguments for medical nihilism.

What about alternative medicine? Many people use alternative medicine, such as homeopathy and acupuncture, in the hope that it will improve their health. Is there anything to be said in favor of this? A straightforward dismissive answer notes that the vast majority of trials that have tested alternative medicine show it to be no better than placebo, and thus alternative medicine is not effective. However, on the basis of what we have learned about the nature of health and disease, and about how interventions are empirically evaluated, we will see that this dismissive answer is too hasty. The question about the effectiveness of alternative medicine, it turns out, is puzzling. A similar puzzle applies to the notion of placebo. At the end of the chapter we study the notion of placebo and ask whether or not placebos can be deemed effective.

To define effectiveness of medical interventions as the capacity to improve health, perhaps by targeting a disease, is a fine starting point. But as we saw in chapters 1 and 2, by defining effectiveness this way we rely on two thorny notions: health and disease. How we conceive of effectiveness is influenced by how we conceive of health and disease.

For example, suppose we are neutralists about health. On this account, health is just the absence of disease. Since our working definition of effectiveness holds that a medical intervention is effective if it improves health, then, according to neutralism, effective medical interventions can only improve health by eliminating or mitigating diseases (remember that "disease" in this context refers to all ways in which a person can be less than healthy, including injuries). On this way of thinking, a medical intervention cannot be deemed effective if it simply improves functioning beyond that achieved once disease has been eliminated—that is, if it enhances "positive health." So, for example, exogenous growth hormone could be an effective intervention for Sam, who is unusually short due to a growth hormone deficiency, but exogenous growth hormone could not be an effective intervention for Joe, who is of normal height but wants to be taller so he can play professional basketball. (However, this assumes a sharp distinction between treatment and enhancement, and critics like to point out that this distinction is difficult to ground in natural facts. Consider another boy, Mike, who is unusually short because his parents are short—he doesn't have a microphysiological abnormality like Sam does . . . or does he? After all, there is an inherited physical basis to his abnormal height.)

On the other hand, if we hold a positive view of health, like that of the World Health Organization, then medical interventions can be effective in many more ways than merely eliminating or mitigating diseases. Anything that contributes to a person's "state of complete physical, mental and social well-being" can be deemed an effective medical intervention in virtue of its capacity to improve positive health. This notion of effectiveness inherits some difficulties of the positive account of health. All sorts of things can improve a person's physical, mental, and social well-being, such as a nutritious supper, time with loving family, and rewarding hobbies. To call these things "effective medical interventions" is, at the very least, inconsistent with typical linguistic usage.

Similarly, one's conception of disease influences one's conception of effectiveness. Recall the view of disease called naturalism: for a condition to be a disease, according to naturalism, it is necessary that this condition be characterized by abnormal biological functioning. So, according to naturalism, a medical intervention can be effective if it targets that abnormal biological functioning and returns this functioning to normal, or at least closer to normal. For example, exogenously administered insulin is an effective intervention for type 1 diabetes because it makes up for the incapacity of the beta cells of the pancreases of diabetic patients to produce endogenous insulin; this intervention modulates the abnormal physiological functioning that results from a dearth of endogenous insulin.

Alternatively, consider normativism, which holds that for a condition to be a disease, that condition must harm a person who has that condition. So, according to normativism, a medical intervention can be effective if it mitigates the harm caused by a disease. For example, an opiate alleviates the pain of a sore back, and thus is an effective intervention for that sore back even if the opiate does not modulate the constitutive causal basis of the sore back.

Or consider hybridism, which holds that for a condition to be a disease it must be characterized by abnormal biological functioning and cause harm to a person with the condition. Since there are two fundamental aspects to disease, according to hybridism, a medical intervention is effective if it targets at least one of these two aspects. So, according to hybridism, a medical intervention can be effective if it either targets the abnormal biological functioning of a disease and returns this functioning to normal (or at least closer to normal), or if the medical intervention mitigates the harm caused by a disease. The account of effectiveness based on hybridism explains why medicine has the two very fundamental aims of *care* and *cure*: if an intervention targets the harm caused by a disease then it offers some care, and if an intervention targets the abnormal biological functioning of a disease then it goes some way toward cure (though of course the vast majority of medical interventions are a long way from cures).

Many people today operate on the assumption that medical interventions can be, and often are, effective at intervening on diseases. But this assumption was not always so widespread. Consider the following passage:

> I was a medical student at the time of sulfanilamide and penicillin, and I remember the earliest reaction of flat disbelief concerning such things. We had given up on therapy, a century earlier. With a few exceptions which we regarded as anomalies, such as vitamin B for pellagra, liver extract for pernicious anaemia, and insulin for diabetes, we were educated to be skeptical about the treatment of disease. Miliary tuberculosis and subacute bacterial endocarditis were fatal in 100 percent of cases, and we were convinced that the course of master diseases like these could never be changed, not in our lifetime or in any other. Overnight we became optimists, enthusiasts. The realisation that disease could be turned around by treatment, provided that one knew enough about the underlying mechanism, was a totally new idea just forty years ago.
> —Lewis Thomas (cited in Bluhm and Borgerson)

So, before the advent of antibiotics and a few successful interventions like insulin for type 1 diabetes, many physicians held modest views about the effectiveness of their therapeutic arsenal. We will examine this skeptical position in the next section. In any case, today many people expect medical interventions to be effective. Of course, medical interventions are not thought of as either effective or ineffective, but rather as effective to some degree. That is, effectiveness is a property to be measured. This raises the question we studied in chapters 7 and 9: How ought the effectiveness of medical interventions be measured?

10.3 MEDICAL NIHILISM

Medicine has always had its critics. Even Hippocrates, the symbolic forebear of modern medicine, was critical of medical practice and clinical treatments, and held that not intervening at all was often the best way to treat patients. In early modern European culture, medicine was highly distrusted. Shakespeare, for example, had one of his characters say, "Trust not the physician; His antidotes are poison, and he slays" (*Timon of Athens*). Centuries later, in the middle of the nineteenth century, Oliver Wendell Holmes Sr., who was at the time the dean of the Harvard Medical School, wrote, "If the whole materia medica, as now used, could be sunk to the bottom of the sea, it would be all the better for mankind—and all the worse for the fishes." Medicine went through a golden age of discoveries starting at the end of the nineteenth century and for several decades after. There were theoretical developments (such as the germ theory of disease), methodological developments (such as the development of modern statistics), and therapeutic developments (such as the discovery of antibiotics).

Even after this renaissance in medical research and practice, there are prominent critics of medicine today. These include some well-known epidemiologists (such as John Ioannidis, who in a famous article argued that most published research findings are false), physicians (such as Marcia Angell, the former editor of one of the world's most important medical journals, who claimed that very few new drugs are beneficial), and philosophers (who articulate worries about the methods of medical research, as discussed in chapter 7, for example, and the theoretical presuppositions underlying many medical interventions). Consider this: Richard Smith, the former editor of the *British Medical Journal*, and so surely someone who has an insider's insight into contemporary medicine, wrote that if someone is dying from cancer they could make the death bearable with "love, morphine, and whisky," but they ought to avoid "overambitious oncologists."

The skepticism about medicine in the nineteenth century, represented by the passage from Holmes, was referred to as *therapeutic nihilism*. Because the skepticism about medicine today is about more features of medicine than therapy, I prefer the term *medical nihilism* to refer to this cluster of skeptical positions. What justifies these skeptics? What are the arguments that these critics raise for medical nihilism?

Some epidemiologists and physicians point to empirical data. Since roughly the start of the twenty-first century, methods like randomized trials and meta-analyses show that medical interventions, on average, have very small effect sizes. Others point to problems with the research methods themselves, arguing that trials and meta-analyses can be unreliable for the reasons we saw in chapter 7, and these problems usually bias methods toward overestimating the effectiveness of interventions and underestimating their harms. Others note finergrained technical problems with contemporary medical research, pertaining to fundamental issues in statistics and trial design. Others worry about the social context in which medical research is carried out, noting that most trials are performed and analyzed by the companies who manufacture the products being tested by those trials; this is a conflict of interest that can exacerbate the methodological problems of medical research (chapter 8).

Still others argue that our theoretical understanding of many diseases and the interventions for those diseases is very poor, which mitigates our ability to effectively intervene on such diseases. Some critics argue that many alleged diseases today are not genuine diseases, and thus we ought not be attempting to use medicine to intervene on them in the first place. In short, arguments for medical nihilism draw on numerous problems in medicine, many of which we study in this book. It is a position that I myself am sympathetic with, and I wrote a book in which I explore many of the above arguments in detail.

One conclusion of the arguments for medical nihilism is that medical interventions, on average, are not nearly as effective as many people think. There are many prominent examples. Consider SSRIs, which are a class of "antidepressants." Recent meta-analyses suggest that these drugs are hardly better than placebo at lowering symptoms of depression, and are often quite harmful. Or consider drugs like statins, which are widely prescribed to lower cholesterol levels in the hope of mitigating the risk of heart attack and death. Physicians have to give about 60 people who have had no history of heart disease statins for five years in order to avoid a single nonfatal heart attack, and in this population statins do not decrease mortality; conversely, statins cause significant harms, such as muscle damage and diabetes.

In addition to many examples of medical interventions that appear to have low effectiveness, medicine also appears to have little ability to predict. Prognosis is a prediction about how a patient will do given some course of treatment. Consider some examples. A woman with stage 1 breast cancer: Will she be alive in five years? Will her cancer reappear if she takes tamoxifen? A man with depression: Will this antidepressant lower his self-reported symptoms? A man with high cholesterol: Will he suffer a heart attack within the next five years? A psychotic patient admitted to a clinic, currently on five prescription drugs and one recreational drug: Will taking him off two of the prescription drugs make him better or worse? These are all bread-and-butter examples from contemporary medicine; the diseases are among the most frequently diagnosed. The honest answer to all these prognostic questions is that we don't know. Medicine is not very good at predicting patient outcomes (for all but a few diseases and treatments).

Many people are drawn to skepticism about medicine because of their suspicions regarding the role of private industry in medicine. We saw some of the nefarious influences that the pharmaceutical industry has on medical research in chapter 8. The worry, arguably justified, is that the great financial stakes for pharmaceutical companies create conflicts of interest when it comes to studying their own products. These conflicts of interest render the research that is funded and controlled by pharmaceutical companies untrustworthy, goes this worry.

How should this general skeptical position be evaluated? Is medical nihilism a compelling thesis? One puzzling question that arises is this: If medicine has been so bad at achieving its goals of curing diseases and caring for patients, how has it managed to maintain such prestige over the millennia? Of course, medicine is a highly revered profession (as suggested by the rigorous education of medical students and the high salaries of medical professionals). What can explain the apparent contrast between the arguments for medical nihilism and the prestige that we readily grant medicine? These are interesting and provocative questions, but we will not dwell on them here. Instead, we will turn to other provocative topics.

After learning about medical nihilism above, you might think that, on the basis of the skepticism that medical nihilism fosters, we ought to be using more "alternative medicine." Or, you might think that the arguments that motivate medical nihilism apply to alternative medicine even more strongly. What is alternative medicine? Is it a compelling way to improve our health?

Alternative medicine is a system of delivering interventions, and sometimes of conceiving of diseases, that are not deemed part of mainstream Western medicine. Such practices include homeopathy, acupuncture, and reiki. Here is a definition of "complementary and alternative medicine" offered by the National Institutes of Health: "a group of diverse medical and health care systems, practices, and products that are not presently considered to be part of conventional medicine." This definition leaves a lot to quibble about, but let's jump straight to the substantive issues. People spend many billions of dollars every year on alternative medicine, and sometimes forego mainstream medicine while using alternative medicine. Alternative medicine sharply divides many people into two camps: critics and defenders. Critics claim that alternative medicine has not been rigorously tested and is based on dubious theoretical presuppositions. Defenders defend. How should we assess this dispute? Is alternative medicine effective? How should this be tested?

There are two fundamental points of dispute between critics and defenders of alternative medicine: one about evidence and the other about theory. Let's look at each dispute in turn.

The evidential dispute about alternative medicine hinges on what one takes to be the appropriate evidential standard for testing alternative medicine. Defenders argue that many millions of people report improved health thanks to alternative medicines. Since these practices have been around for many centuries, and so many people claim to have benefited from them, the empirical basis for the effectiveness of alternative medicines is strong, claim the defenders. Critics argue that this empirical basis, no matter how large or longstanding, is shot through with the various biases we learned about in chapter 7, including confirmation bias, exacerbated by the natural course of diseases. Critics argue that when alternative medicine is tested according to the standards of mainstream medicine, designed to avoid such biases, alternative medicine appears ineffective. We saw in chapter 7 that the evidence-based medicine standard for testing the effectiveness of interventions is the randomized trial and meta-analyses of such trials. When practices like homeopathy are tested by randomized trials, they usually appear ineffective.

In response, defenders argue that the setting of randomized trials is excessively artificial and cannot incorporate the full range of activities and expertise that constitutes alternative medicines. Practices like reiki and acupuncture, for example, are not as simple as giving a patient a pill. The basic thrust of this defense is to appeal to the holistic nature of alternative medicine interventions: the efficacy of an alternative medicine intervention is not due to one single aspect of the intervention, but rather is due to the whole package of aspects of the intervention, including the careful and attentive relationship between provider and patient. So, to determine the effectiveness of a homeopathic remedy by isolating the causal "substance" and administering it in a controlled, double-blinded, randomized trial would be to leave out most of what makes homeopathy effective (goes this defense).

Critics remain unimpressed by this. There is no reason, in principle, why the holistic nature of the treatment itself cannot be tested, claim critics. Evidence-based medicine uses the term *pragmatic trial* to refer to randomized trials in which an intervention is tested in its natural setting, including the subtle features of the patient-provider interaction. Pragmatic trials, claim critics, can be used to test the holistic nature of alternative medicine.

However, for many alternative medicine modalities, double-blinding is impossible. So a pragmatic trial of such a modality may have the various forms of bias discussed in chapter 7. Thus if a pragmatic trial of an alternative medicine provides evidence that the intervention is effective, that might be a result of the bias and not the true effectiveness of the intervention. Defenders, in turn, reiterate some of the arguments for medical nihilism discussed in the previous section: research testing many mainstream medical interventions also has many biases. For instance, in trials of antidepressants, subjects frequently are able to guess whether or not they are in the intervention group or the control group (on the basis of what sorts of side effects they experience), and thus these trials also end up being unblinded. Defenders conclude that it is unfair to judge the empirical basis of alternative medicine on the grounds that this empirical basis is biased, because the empirical basis of mainstream medicine is also biased. Of course, if you are swayed by the arguments for medical nihilism then you will be unconvinced by this rejoinder (since you might end up thinking that both mainstream medicine and alternative medicine are to be regarded with a healthy dose of skepticism).

Defenders also articulate challenges to the very principles of evidence-based medicine. Recall in chapter 7 the critiques of randomized trials and meta-analyses. A strong conclusion from these critiques would be that the set of epistemological principles employed to assess medical interventions is itself unfounded. If so, then one cannot criticize alternative medicine on the grounds that it does not satisfy the evidential standards of evidence-based medicine. Supposing this line of reasoning were compelling, defenders of alternative medicine would be on sturdier footing regarding the evidential basis of alternative medicine. However, a more modest conclusion from the critiques of the set of epistemological principles of evidence-based medicine would be to admit that randomized trials and meta-analyses are fallible, that mechanistic knowledge should be incorporated into inferences regarding effectiveness of interventions, and more care should be taken with the statistical aspects of such inferences, but nevertheless that this cluster of methods is the best we have to go on when it comes to assessing the effectiveness of interventions. On these grounds, alternative medicine does not seem very compelling.

Critics and defenders of alternative medicine also disagree on its theoretical basis. Critics argue that the purported theoretical underpinnings of alternative medicine interventions are inconsistent with well-established physical, chemical, and biological theories. If one of these alternative medicine theories were correct, then some extremely important scientific theories would have to be false. But on the basis of everything we know, including our very best scientific research, these scientific theories are true, or at least approximately true. Therefore, the purported theoretical underpinnings of alternative medicine are false. For example, homeopathy involves diluting substances in water over and over again, until there is virtually none of the original substance left in the water. Homeopaths claim that water retains a memory of diluted substances, which they claim is responsible for the alleged effects of homeopathy. But after centuries of careful study of the chemistry of water, nearly no reputable scientist believes that water has such a memory.

Conversely, defenders of alternative medicine argue that Western medicine is excessively committed to reductionist thinking, whereas alternative medicine is holistic—this is pertinent not just to the appropriate methodology for testing alternative medicine interventions, as above, but also to assessing the theoretical basis of alternative medicine (chapter 5). The mistake that critics make, according to this line of reasoning, is to think that alternative medicine must be understood in terms that are familiar to Western medicine, which involves conceiving of diseases in microphysiological terms and formulating interventions that target those microphysiological features. Alternative medicine, defenders argue, is about more than the reductionist basis of disease; it is about the whole life of a patient, including elements of one's lifestyle, such as diet, exercise, stress, and relationships, that influence one's well-being. Defenders hold that these broader features of one's life are often the root cause of diseases, and thus it is these features that should be targeted by intervention—mainstream medicine, goes this line of reasoning, too often targets symptoms of disease rather than the deep causes. Moreover, defenders of alternative medicine claim that mainstream medical interventions are often toxic. The French term for alternative medicine is "médecine douce," which can be translated as "gentle medicine"—this represents a view of defenders that alternative medicines have fewer side effects than mainstream medical interventions, and thus do less harm.

Given the constraints on testing alternative medicine, and given quite a lot of evidence from randomized trials, the effectiveness of most alternative medicine interventions appears little different than placebo. Such, anyway, is the main complaint of the critics. The worry that the placebo effect accounts for much of the effectiveness of interventions is also a main argument for skepticism about mainstream medicine. So, in the next section we examine the placebo effect.

10.5 PLACEBO

Most of us are familiar with the general idea of the placebo effect. Merely by consuming what we think is a medical intervention, and being attended to by healthcare workers, we have a tendency to feel better. The misattribution of the efficacy of the placebo effect to the intervention is exacerbated by the natural course of many diseases, in which symptoms can diminish over time without any intervention at all. In chapter 7 we studied the role of expectation bias and features of trial design intended to minimize expectation bias. Here we directly examine placebos. What exactly is a placebo? Can we consider placebos to be effective? Should physicians use placebos in clinical practice?

The point of comparing the effects of an experimental intervention in one group with the effects of a control intervention in a control group is to determine the effects of the experimental intervention that go beyond what would happen to subjects without any intervention. The point of using placebos as the control intervention is to attempt to determine the effects of an experimental intervention that go beyond the effects that would be elicited in subjects merely due to the fact that they are receiving some sort of care from a physician, due to their expectations of improvement.

Placebos are often thought of as inert substances, in contrast with pharmacologically active substances in drugs. Yet placebos are employed in clinical research precisely because they elicit physiological effects, so in a straightforward sense they cannot be inert. It is flirting with contradiction to say that a physiologically inert substance can elicit physiological effects. Moreover, whether or not a substance is inert depends in part on the condition being intervened upon: a sugar pill, for example, will not be inert for a patient with diabetes. Indeed, inert substances can make for a bad placebo, as we will see below.

Instead, another way to define placebos is simply by reference to expectation effects. Both physicians and patients have expectations that arise from the administration of an intervention. This usually involves expectations of the patient improving, but can also involve expectations that the patient will experience particular side effects. There is a large amount of evidence that such expectations (either the physician's expectations, or the patient's, or both) can actually cause physical changes in the patient: the severity of a patient's symptoms can decrease, for example, merely as a result of expecting her symptoms to decrease. One of the most prominent sources of such expectations is the administration of an intervention. This is not the only source of such expectations—for instance, you might have an expectation that the symptoms of your cold will improve over time because you know that this is what typically occurs—but the administration of an intervention is an important source of such expectations. The use of placebo controls in a randomized trial is meant to ensure that whatever expectation effects that arise from the administration of the intervention are elicited in both the intervention group and the comparison (or "control") group. Placebos are interventions that elicit effects in people via expectations.

Precisely how expectation effects occur is mysterious. That is, we do not understand the mechanism by which expectation effects arise. Nevertheless, it is reasonable to assume that there is such a mechanism (or set of mechanisms), and indeed, much research today is designed to better understand the mechanisms by which placebos elicit effects.

Interventions can elicit effects in people both via "pharmacological" mechanisms and via expectation mechanisms. In short, pharmacological mechanisms are the specific biochemical entities and pathways that are modulated by interventions: drugs typically function as ligands, which bind to receptors and modulate their activity, which thereby modulate one or more biochemical pathways, which elicits physiological responses. Thus we might think that expectation effects can be understood as the physiological (or psychological) changes in a patient that (i) occur after consuming an intervention,

(ii) are not a result of the pharmacological mechanisms, and (iii) would not have occurred without the intervention.

But expectation effects are even more complicated than this. For instance, expectation effects can arise as a result of pharmacological effects. Suppose that an experimental drug for depression is thought to have two prominent and harmful side effects: weight gain and diminished interest in sex. Subjects who are recruited into a trial to test this drug are told that this is a risk of the drug (a necessary condition to get proper consent from subjects is to inform them of the potential risks of participating in the trial). A particular subject in the trial is not told which group she is in (the experimental drug group or the placebo group), but she in fact is in the experimental group. After a couple of weeks into the trial she begins to gain weight and lose interest in sex. As a result, she guesses that she is in the intervention group, and she thereby generates an expectation that her depression will be helped. Thus, an expectation effect is generated by a result of the pharmacological effects (in this case, the side effects) of the drug.

This phenomenon is a widespread problem in clinical research. Subjects are often able to guess what group of a trial they are in. This is "blind breaking" (because the blinding of the subject regarding which group she is in has been "broken"). This is a problem precisely because of the expectation effects that can arise once a subject knows (or is able to guess) if she is receiving the experimental intervention or a placebo. For this reason, placebos are often designed to elicit physiological responses that mimic, as much as possible, the experimental intervention being tested in its profile of side effects. But even with such placebos, subjects are often able to accurately guess what group of a trial they are in. Occasionally trials are designed such that subjects are asked to guess what trial they are in, so that researchers can make estimates of the frequency of blind breaking (this is not done on a routine basis, but arguably should be).

There are two additional nuances about expectation effects that we should be aware of. The first is that some diseases are more "placebo responsive" than other diseases. For many psychiatric diseases, for example, the expectation effects of placebos can be very large, whereas for a disease such as type 1 diabetes, the expectation effects of placebos are much smaller (if you have type 1 diabetes, it's hard to fool your pancreas into producing insulin).

The second is that not all expectation effects are beneficial for a patient. The term *nocebo effect* refers to expectation effects that are detrimental to a person's health. Think of the example above, in which an experimental drug for depression has two harmful side effects: weight gain and diminished interest in sex. Suppose after a couple of weeks into the trial, a subject in the placebo group gains a little weight, and she wrongly guesses that she is in the intervention group, which leads her to generate an expectation that she will suffer from the other side effect, namely, a diminished interest in sex.

Most expectation effects, as far as we know, are beneficial—most are not nocebo, but placebo. Can medicine harness this power of expectation effects to improve people's health? In a sense, medicine already incorporates expectation effects. As we noted above, medical interventions elicit effects via two sets of mechanisms: the active pharmacological mechanisms and the expectation mechanisms. Medical interventions operate via both kinds of mechanisms, and thus medicine already harnesses expectation effects. However, one of the criticisms of mainstream medicine is that many contemporary medical interventions are very toxic and are not much better than placebo (which operates via expectation mechanisms). So, one possibility could be to use interventions that do not operate via pharmacological mechanisms but only via expectation mechanisms. In other words, medicine could use placebos. Since we know placebos can elicit significant beneficial effects, typically without the harmful side effects of drugs, placebos can be very good for people. Should medicine use placebos to treat people?

One answer to this question is, straightforwardly, yes. According to this view, physicians ought to prescribe placebos to their patients, even if this involves deceiving their patients. After all, placebos do little harm but can do plenty of good. Let's call this view *paternalism* about placebos. Conversely, another possible answer is, straightforwardly, no. According to this view, physicians ought to respect the autonomy of their patients, which involves being honest with them. Lying, on this view, amounts to taking away the possibility of a patient freely choosing for oneself. One's view about placebo paternalism might depend in part on one's broader view about lying, and perhaps on one's more fundamental view on the foundations of ethics: if you are inclined toward consequentialism then you might think paternalism about placebos is fine (since deceptive use of placebos can cause good consequences), whereas if you are inclined toward a principled non-consequentialist ethics then you might think paternalism about placebos is not okay (since on such a view deception generally is not okay).

However, there might be a middle position on placebo paternalism. Recent research suggests that people can be placebo-responsive even when they know they are receiving a placebo. It might sound strange. But if this phenomenon is true, then medicine could employ placebos (at least in some circumstances) without deceiving patients.

FURTHER READING

Defining effectiveness: Stegenga (2015b)

Medical nihilism: Illich (1975), Stegenga (2018), Wootton (2006), Ioannidis (2005)

Alternative medicine: Borgerson (2005)

Placebo: Holman (2015), Howick (2017)

DISCUSSION QUESTIONS

1. What must a medical intervention do in order for that intervention to be deemed effective?
2. What does medical nihilism entail for one of the following: clinical practice, the biomedical research agenda, methodological standards, regulation, or intellectual property laws?
3. Should doctors prescribe placebos to their patients?
4. Is contemporary medical research reliable? Explain.

11 : DIAGNOSIS AND SCREENING

11.1 SUMMARY

Diagnosis has received less philosophical scrutiny than other aspects of medicine, though recently there has been some critical discussion of diagnosis, screening, and related problems, such as "overdiagnosis." Diagnosis involves the consideration of a range of signs, symptoms, background information about patients, and results of diagnostic tests, in order to infer whether or not a person has a particular disease. Some philosophers have argued that diagnosis is a good illustration of "inference to the best explanation": to make a diagnosis a physician must offer the best explanation of the various signs and symptoms of the patient, and such explanations typically take the form of positing the presence of a particular disease in a patient.

Though diagnosis in general has received little discussion from philosophers, the probabilistic nature of diagnostic tests has long served as an illustration of inductive reasoning for theories of statistical inference. This chapter describes some of the core logical features underlying medical tests. A medical test is designed to provide evidence regarding whether or not a person has a particular disease: a positive test result for disease d suggests that a person has d, while a negative test result suggests that a person does not have d. However, such tests are fallible. Sometimes a test suggests that a person has d when they do not in fact have d (this is called a *false positive*), and sometimes a test suggests that a person does not have d when they do in fact have d (this is called a *false negative*). False positives and false negatives can have serious practical consequences. False positives can lead to needless stress and anxiety and sometimes needless treatments, while false negatives can lead to people foregoing potentially helpful treatments.

Screening involves the routine administration of diagnostic tests to asymptomatic people in an attempt to find diseases at earlier rather than later stages. There are vigorous debates about whether or not particular kinds of people should be actively screened for particular diseases. For example, should women under the age of fifty receive regular mammograms? Like the argument from inductive risk, there are practical consequences of both too much screening and too little screening. Too much screening can lead to false positives, more invasive forms of screening such as biopsies, "overdiagnosis," and subsequently "overtreatment." Too little screening has the opposite problem: it can lead to "underdiagnosis" and hence "undertreatment." We will study some aspects of these debates in this chapter.

11.2 DIAGNOSIS

Before developing a treatment plan or offering a prognosis to a patient, a physician usually must develop a diagnosis. There are several interesting philosophical questions about diagnosis.

The main point of diagnosis is, of course, to establish what disease a patient has. The evidence that physicians appeal to in order to make a diagnosis includes patient symptoms and laboratory tests, and can also include broader features of a patient's life. For instance, suppose a patient tells a physician that she is suffering from fever, chills, muscle aches, and joint pain. The physician might initially infer that the patient has influenza. That would explain these symptoms. However, suppose the patient tells the physician that five days ago she was hiking in the woods, and two days after the hike she found a tick on her leg. The physician might now infer that, rather than influenza, the patient has Lyme disease. That's because, although the hiking and the tick are not strictly speaking symptoms, they are clues that the symptoms are not caused by influenza but rather by the bacteria that is spread by ticks and is the constitutive causal basis of Lyme disease.

We saw in chapter 4 (§4.4) that there are several ways of formulating a system of disease classification. Nosology can be based on the etiology of diseases, on the pathophysiology of diseases, or on the symptoms of diseases. Notice, though, that diagnosis is, obviously, itself based on symptoms of diseases. If a disease definition is based on symptoms, and a person satisfies the symptom-based diagnostic criteria for that disease, then that person, by definition, has the disease. I discuss this strange aspect of symptom-based nosology in the chapter on psychiatry (chapter 12), because psychiatry employs a symptom-based nosology.

Diagnoses are often thought to be *explanations*, specifically causal explanations. That is, a diagnosis is an inference to the best explanation of the cause or causes of symptoms. For example, if a patient has chest pain and a bad cough for three weeks, and a laboratory test indicates an infection with *Mycobacterium tuberculosis*, the diagnosis "tuberculosis" explains the symptoms—the presence of the bacterium explains why the patient suffers chest pain and has a cough. Some diagnoses, however, are not very explanatory. Idiopathic diseases are those for which we do not know what the underlying constitutive causal basis is. For example, ankylosing spondylitis is a form of arthritis which is characterized by inflammation of the joints of the spine. Symptoms include joint stiffness and back pain. A diagnosis of ankylosing spondylitis offers little more than a redescription of that which a patient suffers from. Critics of psychiatry claim that most psychiatric diagnoses are not explanatory at all, because they are entirely redescriptions of symptoms—as noted above and in more detail in chapter 12, psychiatric nosology is symptom-based, and thus a psychiatric diagnosis cannot explain the symptoms.

One might deny that diagnoses are meant to be explanatory. One could be strictly pragmatic about diagnosis. On this view, a diagnosis does not have to postulate a causal explanation of symptoms. Instead, a diagnosis merely must offer a label that can be used to communicate with patients and colleagues, teach medical students, and justify treatment decisions. These are important ends that a diagnosis can satisfy, even if the diagnosis is not explanatory. On this view, there would be nothing wrong with a symptom-based diagnosis, such as is used in psychiatry, as long as a particular diagnosis can in fact satisfy these other ends. When it comes to explaining the presence of a disease, we saw in chapter 5 that there is a key division between holism and reductionism: holism says that we should explain diseases by understanding the whole context of a patient's condition, including facts about their life, their history, their family, and so on, while reductionism says that we should explain diseases by understanding the microphysiological causes of the symptoms of the disease.

Another question about diagnosis is this: How should diagnostic tests be evaluated? In the next section (§11.3) we will examine the underlying logic of diagnostic tests. We will see that a premise of the logic of diagnostic tests is knowledge about the accuracy of tests. We will examine precisely what accuracy means for diagnostic tests in §11.3. A related question is how to estimate the accuracy of diagnostic tests. We saw in earlier chapters that medical scientists consider the randomized trial to be the best method for testing the effectiveness of medical interventions (though we also saw that this is challenged by critics). Randomized trials are now sometimes used to evaluate the accuracy of diagnostic tests. In any case, to evaluate the accuracy of a diagnostic test, it must be compared with a "gold standard" test.

There are some diagnostic tests for diseases that cannot be treated, such as a genetic test that predicts Huntington's disease. Are these tests valuable, despite the fact that we cannot do anything once we have the results of the tests? Some people say no. Since medicine is an applied science, diagnostic tests should be performed only if we can take action based on the results of those tests. Other people say yes. Merely knowing about one's physiological condition, regardless of whether or not one can do anything about that condition, can be valuable for some people.

11.3 LOGIC OF DIAGNOSTIC TESTS

Some medical tests are measurements of continuous physiological parameters, such as blood pressure or hormone levels. Other medical tests provide indications regarding whether or not a binary physiological parameter is present, such as being infected with the bacterium *Mycobacterium tuberculosis*, being pregnant, having cancer, or having a broken bone. To understand the logic of medical tests, we will focus on tests for binary physiological parameters.

A test for the presence of disease d can return two values. Let's call these values + (the test indicates that the disease is present) and − (the test indicates that the disease is absent). Because the physiological property is deemed to be binary, there are two possible true states: having the disease (d) and not having the disease ($\sim d$). So there are four possible combinations of the indication of the test and the state of the person being tested:

- $+$ & d: the test indicates the presence of the disease, and the person has the disease ("true positive")
- $+$ & $\sim d$: the test indicates the presence of the disease, but the person does not have the disease ("false positive")
- $-$ & d: the test indicates the absence of the disease, but the person has the disease ("false negative")
- $-$ & $\sim d$: the test indicates the absence of the disease, and the person does not have the disease ("true negative")

So there are two ways that a diagnostic test can be accurate, and two ways a diagnostic test can be inaccurate. The "sensitivity" of a diagnostic test is the "true positive" rate of a test: the proportion of true cases of the presence of disease that are accurately identified as cases of disease. Sensitivity is the complement to the "false negative" rate: the proportion of true positive cases of disease that are inaccurately identified as not being cases of disease. Thus, sensitivity equals one minus the false negative rate. The "specificity" of a diagnostic test is the "true negative" rate of a test: the proportion of true cases of absence of disease that are accurately identified as cases in which there is no disease. Specificity is the complement to the "false positive" rate: the proportion of cases of absence of diseases that are inaccurately identified as cases of disease. Thus, specificity equals one minus the false positive rate.

Diagnosis involves a physician determining how likely it is that d—that is, what the probability is that the person has the disease. Of course, diagnosis can be aided with the results of screening tests. If a test returns a $+$ indication, this increases the probability that d is the case. Upon receiving a positive test result, the physician must estimate the probability that d, given the test result. It turns out that most people, including physicians, are not very good at such estimations.

Consider a screening test which is very accurate. Its sensitivity is 99%: if a person has the disease (that is, if d) then the test indicates $+$ 99% of the time, and so its false negative rate is 1%. Its specificity is

98%: if a person does not have the disease (that is, if ~d) then the test indicates – 98% of the time, and so its false positive rate is 2%. If a person is screened with the test and the test indicates +, what is the probability that the person has the disease? Many people jump to the conclusion that the answer is 99%, or maybe 98%, or some other high probability. The problem with such an answer is that it is another instance of the base-rate fallacy, which we learned about in chapter 9. We cannot answer the question as it is stated because we do not have enough information. The question is about a conditional probability: the probability that a person has the disease given that the test indicates that they have the disease. Using our notation, the question is about the probability that d, given +. More formally: what is P(d|+)?

So the question boils down to determining a conditional probability. We learned in chapter 9 that there is a handy formula for calculating conditional probabilities: Bayes' Theorem. That is:

$$P(d|+) = P(+|d)P(d)/[P(+|d)P(d) + P(+|{\sim}d)P({\sim}d)]$$

Once we translate these terms into plain language we'll see that this math is pretty simple.

The first term on the left side of the equation, P(d|+), is the probability that a person has the disease given that the test indicates that they have the disease—this is what the physician wants to determine. The first term on the right side of the equation, P(+|d), is the probability that the test would indicate that a person has a disease given the the person in fact has the disease—this is the true positive rate, which we know is 99%, or a probability of .99. The next term, P(d), is the prior probability that the person has the disease, or the base-rate of the disease. This is the key piece of information that was missing in the original description of the problem. We need to know this quantity in order to answer the physician's question. Let's suppose that the disease occurs once in every 5000 people. Then P(d) is 1/5000, or 0.0002. The penultimate remaining term in the formula, P(+|~d), is the probability that the test would indicate that a person has a disease given that the person does not have the disease—this is the false positive rate, which we know is 2%, or a probability of 0.02. The final term in the formula, P(~d), is the prior probability that a person does not have the disease, which is 4999/5000 or 0.9998. Now we are ready to determine the probability that a person who tests positive for the disease in fact has the disease. Let's plug the values into the formula:

$$P(d|+) = (0.99)(0.0002)/[(0.99)(0.0002) + (0.02)(0.9998)]$$
$$= 0.0098$$

This rounds up to 0.01. In other words, given that the test indicates that this person has the disease, the probability that a person in fact has the disease is only 0.01. There is only a 1% chance that the person has the disease after getting a positive indication on this test.

The reason this probability is so much lower than the true positive rate and true negative rate (and chances are that it is lower than your initial guess was, too) is because the base-rate or prior probability of the disease in this case was so low. This illustrates how crucially important it is for a physician to take the base-rate of a disease into account when making a diagnosis on the basis of the results of a screening test.

11.4 SCREENING

Screening programs involve actively seeking out cases of diseases. Just like diagnosis, screening involves the use of tests to help determine the chance that a person has a disease. But unlike typical cases of diagnosis, which involve a patient seeking medical attention because of noticeable symptoms, screening involves the active hunt for diseases in a defined population whether or not members of that population have noticeable symptoms. For example, many women over the age of fifty are routinely screened for breast cancer with mammograms (x-rays of the breast); the vast majority of such women do not have symptoms of breast cancer. The reasoning is that routine mammograms in non-symptomatic women can aid in the early detection and diagnosis of breast cancer before the cancer becomes more severe.

Many argue that we should be screening people as actively as we can, in order to detect diseases as early as possible. Early detection permits monitoring and possibly intervention, in order to decrease the possibility of the worsening of a disease. Since some diseases tend to progress from less severe to more severe, the idea behind screening is to identify diseases early so that physicians can monitor their progression and intervene when necessary. Since many cases of early-diagnosed, treatable diseases would otherwise be lethal, screening programs can save many lives. This is the optimistic view on screening.

The pessimistic view on screening is that it can lead to "overdiagnosis." Overdiagnosis occurs when a person is accurately diagnosed with the pathophysiological basis of a disease, but that pathophysiology would never in the life of the patient cause any symptoms. If such a patient were treated for the disease, it becomes a case of overtreatment. Screening programs can lead to overdiagnosis and overtreatment: screening can find real cases of the pathophysiological basis of a disease that otherwise would have gone entirely unnoticed by the patient had they not been screened, because the patient remains asymptomatic. This is especially relevant for elderly patients near the end of their lives, who are very likely to die of causes other than the diagnosed disease. Indeed, one source of evidence for the frequency of overdiagnosis comes from autopsies, which can find the pathophysiological basis of asymptomtatic "diseases," such as benign cancers.

I use the scare quotes around diseases above so that we do not beg the question—recall from chapter 2 that normativism and hybridism about disease require that a condition cause a person harm in order for that condition to be deemed a disease, and thus non-symptomatic physiological abnormalities would not be cases of genuine disease. These cases might seem dangerous but in fact be harmless, such as benign growths that would never actually harm the person. But because of the chance that the abnormal physiological condition could worsen, many patients decide to intervene on it, and so a condition is treated that never would have hurt the patient. Thus the patient is overtreated.

For example, most prostate cancers grow slowly, and thus many men with prostate cancer never experience real harms from the cancer—they do not notice symptoms. However, prostate cancer has become frequently diagnosed and treated (at least in North America) due to the widespread screening with the prostate-specific antigen test (PSA). But critics claim that for most men treated for prostate cancer their quality of life has not improved. Many men treated this way would not have experienced symptoms if they had not been treated, but treatment for prostate cancer can have terrible side effects. So, the use of this screening test, claim critics, contributes to overdiagnosis (and overtreatment).

There is another factor about screening that can contribute to a related problem. As we saw above, in the section on "logic of diagnostic tests," even for excellent screening tests—tests with very low false positive and false negative rates—if the disease being screened for is rare, then the vast majority of people who test positive for the disease will not in fact have the disease. This increases the risk of false positives. Above we studied an example in which a screening test had very low error rates, for a disease which occurs in 1 in 5000 people: for this test, if the result is positive then there is nevertheless only a 1% chance that the person tested actually has the disease. Thus, if people are diagnosed with the disease in question as a result of testing positive on the screening test, then 99% of diagnoses would be false positives. Of course, in most cases physicians base their diagnoses on much more than simply the results of a single test—additional diagnostic information includes symptoms, family history, knowledge of risk factors, and the results of independent tests—but nevertheless this extreme example shows how screening tests can contribute to false positives.

There are other features of medicine that can contribute to overdiagnosis, including the phenomenon of medicalization (which we learned about in chapter 6) and institutional features of healthcare systems. If normal states become medicalized and spurious disease categories are constructed, then more people will be inappropriately diagnosed with a disease, and some of those diagnosed will be inappropriately treated. A related factor that contributes to overdiagnosis is the broadening of disease categories. Typically, for a patient to be diagnosed with a disease they must meet certain requirements—their blood pressure or cholesterol levels have to be above a certain value, for example. When those requirements become easier to satisfy— say, by lowering the threshold for a measured physical parameter to be deemed symptomatic—then the disease category is broadened because more people will satisfy the requirements and thus be diagnosable with the disease. If the disease category is broadened too far—say, by incorporating thresholds for measured physical parameters that are not markers of a genuine disease—then the broadened disease category will contribute to overdiagnosis.

The institutional and legal context of medical practice can also contribute to overdiagnosis and overtreatment. Some physicians feel pressure to diagnose diseases and prescribe treatments out of a concern that if they do not then they are liable to be sued with a malpractice lawsuit. Physicians, moreover, are often paid on a "fee for service" basis that rewards quick turnover of patients, which (so some argue) incentivizes quicker diagnoses and the writing of more prescriptions than they might otherwise write.

To take a controversial example, consider the debate regarding whether or not women in their forties should undergo regular mammogram screening—because of its intensity, this debate has been called the "mammography wars." In a recent review of the available evidence on the benefits and harms of mammography, reviewers concluded that the benefit to women in their forties (that is, a small decrease in mortality caused by breast cancer) does not outweigh the overall costs, which involve radiation exposure, biopsies, and stress—these reviewers do not recommend routine mammograms for women in their forties. Critics of this position, which prominently include professional societies of radiologists (the professional group that provides mammograms), dispute this finding and claim that women in their forties should get routinely screened with mammograms.

In short, the pessimistic view on screening holds that the more we look for diseases, the more cases we will diagnose; some of these cases will be real diseases that would eventually cause harm, while other cases would never cause harm, either because they are false positives or because they are true cases of a physiological abnormality (such as a benign cancerous growth) that will not cause harm.

An objection to the pessimistic view that pro-screeners raise is that many diseases that are screened for can be lethal, and thus even if a screening program has many cases of false positives, which carry the burden of stress and anxiety for those falsely diagnosed, and possibly a burden of overtreatment, identifying the true positive cases is hugely important, because the life of a person properly diagnosed with an otherwise lethal disease can be saved. This is another example of inductive risk in medicine (chapter 8). How one trades off the benefits of routine screening against its harms depends on how one values and disvalues these benefits and harms. Is one life saved worth one thousand unnecessary biopsies? There may be little agreement about such values.

This last point raises another dispute that divides pro-screeners from anti-screeners. How should the benefits of screening programs be measured? One option is to perform trials in which one group of subjects is screened for disease d, another group is not screened for d, and then the number of deaths caused by d in each group is counted and compared—this is to measure "disease-specific mortality." Another option is to perform trials but rather than count only d-caused deaths, count all deaths—this is to measure "all-cause mortality." Which measure should be used in evaluating screening programs: disease-specific mortality or all-cause mortality? The best empirical evaluations of screening programs suggest that some screening programs cause a small decrease in disease-specific mortality, but in these same empirical evaluations there is no difference in all-cause mortality between groups that are screened and groups that are not screened. This is a puzzling phenomenon: the evidence appears to suggest that the very same screening program can lower the number of deaths caused by the disease which is screened for, but not lower the overall number of deaths.

Cynics claim that this is because screening programs themselves cause a slight *increase* in the number of deaths due to causes other than the disease being screened for, thereby offsetting the deaths avoided by the screened disease. Pro-screeners claim that some screening programs do in fact lower all-cause mortality, but because the number of deaths caused by d is a tiny proportion of the overall number of deaths, decreasing d-caused mortality only leads to a tiny decrease in all-cause mortality, and the trials that evaluate screening programs are too small to detect this tiny change in all-cause mortality. Conversely, one might respond by claiming that since screening programs do not have a noticeable effect on all-cause mortality, and ultimately it is living that matters, this is an argument against screening programs.

Notice another feature of screening programs that may trouble you. Most people who undergo screening do not benefit from the screening. Indeed, this is the case for most preventive interventions: the intervention might benefit only one in a hundred, or thousand, people who use it. To use the terminology from chapter 9, the NNT for screening programs is extremely high. We return to this aspect of preventive medicine in chapter 14.

To this, a defender of screening programs could respond by arguing that even though most people who undergo screening do not benefit from it, the few people who do benefit from screening programs achieve great benefits. If a cancer that would have killed a person is detected early enough to remove the cancer, then that person's life is saved or at least prolonged. Since a life saved is such a great outcome, goes this argument, then the small cost to those people who are screened with no benefit is outweighed by the great outcome of a single life saved. How do you think this dispute should be resolved?

FURTHER READING

Diagnosis: Kennedy (2016)
Screening: Plutynski (2012), John (2013), Cassels (2012)
Overdiagnosis: Plutynski (2017)

DISCUSSION QUESTIONS

1. What risks are involved in either under- or over-screening, and how should we balance these risks when making policy?
2. About 1 person in 300 in the USA has HIV. Suppose a person tests positive for HIV based on a diagnostic test with a sensitivity of 99.7% and a specificity of 99.3%, and we know nothing else about this person. What is the probability that the person has HIV, given the positive test result?

3. How should the effectiveness of screening programs be evaluated?
4. Many people take it to be obvious that we should employ disease screening programs to identify cases of disease as early as possible. What reasons have critics articulated against screening programs?

PART IV

Values and Policy

12 : PSYCHIATRY: CARE OR CONTROL?

12.1 SUMMARY

Psychiatry is the branch of medicine that is concerned with diagnosing and treating mental illness, or diseases of the mind. Because the object of psychiatry is the mind, and the many possible troubles of the mind, the theory and practice of psychiatry is extremely complicated and relies on premises of varying philosophical credentials. For this reason, philosophy of psychiatry is its own subdiscipline within philosophy of medicine. As we have seen, there are many philosophical issues in medicine in general, though there is no particular focus on "philosophy of surgery" or "philosophy of dermatology." Philosophy of psychiatry, though, is an active discipline in its own right, and this chapter introduces some of the central questions in this discipline.

There is a sense in which psychiatry is different from the rest of medicine. Certainly the psychiatric disease classification system stands out from the rest of medicine. We saw in chapter 4 that disease classification systems, or nosology, can be based on the etiological causal basis of diseases, the pathophysiological constitutive causal basis of diseases, or the symptoms of diseases. Most of medicine uses one of the first two kinds of classification systems, while psychiatry almost exclusively uses a symptom-based classification system. This is problematic for a number of reasons that we study here.

The title of this chapter gestures toward one of the central debates in philosophy of psychiatry. Some hold that psychiatry is just like the rest of medicine in its ambition: to cure diseases of the mind or at least mitigate the harms caused by diseases of the mind. Critics, on the other hand, hold that psychiatry is very different from the rest of medicine: its function is rather to control deviant behavior. On this account, the ambition of psychiatry is similar to the ambition of legal or religious systems of control: behavior that does not fit with societal norms gets categorized as a disease and controlled with surveillance, with pharmaceuticals, and sometimes even with enforced hospital confinement.

We've already seen philosophical issues about psychiatry in earlier parts of the book, including the section on culture-bound syndromes and the chapter on disease. Here we bring some of these concerns together and focus on several key issues: psychiatric nosology, the anti-psychiatry movement, the nature of delusions, and the justification of context-based diagnostic exclusionary criteria.

12.2 PSYCHIATRIC NOSOLOGY

As we saw in chapter 4, nosology is the part of medicine that focuses on how diseases are defined and categorized. Most of medicine employs pathophysiological or etiological nosology; an example of pathophysiological nosology is the disease category of type 1 diabetes. Psychiatry, however, employs a symptom-based nosology.

Psychiatry became averse to etiological nosology after its earlier use of Freudian etiological theories. In the middle of the twentieth century, psychiatric pathology was explained by reference to Freudian theories, such as poor relationships with one's parents or sexual hangups, but starting with the *DSM-III* (developed in the 1970s and published in 1980), psychiatry eliminated this "theoretical" basis of nosology. Also, because we understand so little about the nature of the mind (either normal or pathological), psychiatry is not in a position to define its diseases in pathophysiological terms. So, because psychiatry dispensed with etiological nosology, and pathophysiological nosology is not at present possible for psychiatry, psychiatric nosology is now based on symptoms alone.

Another motivation for the use of symptom-based nosology was that psychiatry for a long time suffered from a problem of inter-physician reliability. That is, multiple psychiatrists assessing the same person would develop different diagnoses. The developers of *DSM-III* wanted to address this problem of reliability, and so they codified a set of symptom-based diagnoses, which ultimately helped improve reliability. Conversely, however, psychiatric nosology developed a new problem: poor validity. Validity of psychological constructs can mean several different things, but in short, a diagnostic category is valid if it tracks the underlying constitutive or etiological causal basis of the diagnosis. Another way to put the notion of diagnostic validity is that a diagnostic category is valid if it is based on a natural kind. For example, the diagnostic category "tuberculosis" has good validity because all and only people who are accurately diagnosed with tuberculosis have an infection with the bacterium *Mycobacterium tuberculosis*. The symptom-based nosology of psychiatry that was initiated with the *DSM-III* (and that we still use today) explicitly suffers from poor diagnostic validity.

There is something strange about symptom-based nosology: as long as a diagnosis follows standard diagnostic guidelines, a diagnosis cannot be incorrect. Psychiatric practice is a little confusing on this point. The *DSM* is, as the name suggests, a diagnostic manual. But it is more than that. The preface of the *DSM-5* notes that the manual "is a classification of mental disorders with associated criteria designed to facilitate more reliable diagnoses of these disorders." Moreover, the *DSM* says that it is a "categorical classification of separate disorders." So the primary psychiatric diagnostic manual is, at the same time, a diagnostic guide *and* a nosological guide. Its rules of diagnosis are, simultaneously, rules of nosology. We will see that this is a strange and unsatisfying feature of psychiatric nosology.

To ground this discussion, let's consider an important example in detail. Major depressive disorder, colloquially known just as "depression," is a widely diagnosed condition. There are nine diagnostic criteria for depression, and a person must have at least five of them to be diagnosed. But moreover, because depression is defined with respect to these diagnostic criteria, a person who is diagnosed with depression in fact has depression by definition.

Here are the diagnostic criteria. Five (or more) of the following symptoms have been present during the same 2-week period and represent a change from previous functioning; at least one of the symptoms is either (1) depressed mood or (2) loss of interest or pleasure:

1. Depressed mood most of the day, nearly every day, as indicated by either subjective report (e.g., feels sad, empty, hopeless) or observation made by others (e.g., appears tearful). (Note: In children and adolescents, can be irritable mood.)

2. Markedly diminished interest or pleasure in all, or almost all, activities most of the day, nearly every day (as indicated by either subjective account or observation.)

3. Significant weight loss when not dieting or weight gain (e.g., a change of more than 5% of body weight in a month), or decrease or increase in appetite nearly every day. (Note: In children, consider failure to make expected weight gain.)

4. Insomnia or hypersomnia nearly every day.

5. Psychomotor agitation or retardation nearly every day (observable by others, not merely subjective feelings of restlessness or being slowed down).

6. Fatigue or loss of energy nearly every day.

7. Feelings of worthlessness or excessive or inappropriate guilt (which may be delusional) nearly every day (not merely self-reproach or guilt about being sick).

8. Diminished ability to think or concentrate, or indecisiveness, nearly every day (either by subjective account or as observed by others).

9. Recurrent thoughts of death (not just fear of dying), recurrent suicidal ideation without a specific plan, or a suicide attempt or a specific plan for committing suicide.

A strange result of this diagnostic criteria is that people with very different sets of symptoms get diagnosed with the same disease. Suppose Sally has symptoms 1 and 3–6, and Irina has symptoms 2 and 6–9. Both Sally and Irina would be diagnosed with depression, despite the fact that they only share symptom 6. It is reasonable to speculate that Sally and Irina do not, in fact, have the same exact disease. Perhaps they have two subtypes of depression, or perhaps they have two completely different diseases. That is because they share only a single symptom, namely, fatigue.

A related problem is called the problem of "comorbidity." Generally comorbidity refers to the state in which a person has more than one disease. There is nothing spooky or mysterious about a person having, say, influenza and bipolar disorder at the same time. However, in psychiatry critics are skeptical about the reported rates of comorbidity.

The issue is that a very large proportion of people who are diagnosed with a psychiatric disease are also diagnosed with another psychiatric disease. For example, in a large survey, over half of the people who were diagnosed with depression also were diagnosed with an anxiety disorder. Skeptics claim that for many such people they do not in fact have multiple psychiatric diseases; the apparent comorbidity in such cases is an artifact of symptom-based psychiatric nosology in which disease categories are not clearly demarcated. Spurious cases of co-morbidity can lead to overtreatment because in such cases psychiatrists often will prescribe medical interventions for both apparent diseases, when in fact the patient has only one disease.

So, psychiatric nosology lumps together people with the same disease category who in fact have very different presentations of symptoms, and psychiatric nosology assigns multiple disease categories to particular individuals who probably do not have multiple diseases. These problems arise because of the poor diagnostic validity of psychiatric nosology. These diagnostic problems, in turn, entail problems for medical science. Medical scientists study various aspects of diseases in all sorts of ways, at all levels from the genetic to the social. But if the set of people categorized with a particular disease is in fact heterogenous with respect to the disease, then the subsequent scientific work based on such sets of people will be corrupted.

For example, scientists want to know if there is a genetic basis of depression. In order to study this, they perform what is called a *genome-wide association study*, which basically looks at the genomes of people diagnosed with depression and compares them with the genomes of people who are not diagnosed with depression, and looks for any patterns or differences. However, if the set of people diagnosed with depression is in fact very heterogeneous regarding their pathophysiology (and genes), then these genome-wide association studies will have a hard time discovering genuine genetic factors associated with depression.

For the above reasons you might be unsatisfied with symptom-based classifications of diseases. Many people think that psychiatry should define its diseases in the same way that the rest of medicine does. This is the "medical model" of psychiatric nosology. According to the medical model, psychiatry ought to employ either a pathophysiological nosology or an etiological nosology. The medical model holds that psychiatric diseases should be conceived of as diseases of the brain. We should strive to base definitions of psychiatric diseases on physical, brain-based pathologies.

Although psychiatry does not at present define diseases according to pathophysiology, there are numerous pathophysiological theories of psychiatric diseases. Depression is, again, a good example. There are a variety of specific theories about the causes of depression. One such theory was popular for a couple of decades: the monamine theory of depression. This held that depression was caused by an imbalance of neurotransmitters like serotonin. For several empirical and theoretical reasons, the monoamine theory of depression is now not widely accepted among neuroscientists and research psychiatrists.

However, a rejoinder to the demand that psychiatry follow the medical model for nosology is that it might be impossible for psychiatry to do so. Can psychiatric nosology ever be based on anything more than symptoms? Could psychiatric nosology be based on the pathophysiological constitutive basis of diseases? Skeptics say that this would involve solving some of the hard problems in understanding the mind, precisely because mental diseases are disorders of the mind. Psychiatry does have a historically successful precedent of employing the medical model for delineating a disease.

We saw this example in chapter 4. At the end of the nineteenth century the category "psychosis" included all those people who had some form of insanity. But with the rise of germ theory and the discovery that syphilis was caused by a bacterial infection, a subset of psychotic patients was identified as different from the rest. Some patients with psychosis had "neurosyphilis," which is psychosis that is caused by syphilis infection. So, for some cases of psychosis, an etiological cause of their disease was identified. This is taken to be a success story for the possibility of psychiatry to develop from a symptom-based nosology to an etiological or pathophysiological nosology. However, this is a single isolated case, so we ought to be cautious in inferring that most of psychiatry can in fact follow the medical model for nosology.

Here is an exercise designed to illustrate the challenges that symptom-based psychiatric nosology faces, and the fact that symptom-based nosology can be used to pathologize normal aspects of life. Try to guess what normal condition is being referred to in this disease definition. The disease is called Pre-Conscious Hypersomniferosis (PCH). Symptoms include lethargy, changes to eating habits, reduced interest in normal activities, reduced motor activity, occasional hallucinations, diminished sexual activity, and decreased cognitive function. Observed neurological changes include rhythmic electroencephalography patterns and increased blood flow to the brain. The condition has associated endocrine changes, including the release of growth hormone from the pituitary gland. Epidemiological studies show that the severity of the condition is especially high in children and teenagers, but its severity declines in middle adult years. Females have slightly higher rates of this condition than males. There is an inverse correlation between symptom severity and mean income. Patients report that the condition impedes their ability to achieve significant life goals such as the pursuit of career success or the enjoyment of hobbies. This condition responds to pharmacological intervention, especially with stimulants such as caffeine and dextroamphetamine. What normal aspect of life does this alleged disease describe?

12.3 ANTI-PSYCHIATRY

Psychiatry has always had its critics. The content of such criticisms has changed with the changing nature of psychiatry itself, though there have been some general themes that reemerge in different periods.

It's easy to look back on the history of psychiatry with horror. People as far back as 6500 BC practiced trepanation, which involved drilling a hole into a person's skull to release what they thought were evil spirits that caused abnormal behavior. Hydrotherapy was a practice in the early twentieth century—in extreme versions of this form of psychiatric treatment patients were submerged in ice water or restrained in a bath for days at a time. Lobotomy, the discovery of which won the Nobel Prize in 1949, was a widely performed surgery in which the neuronal connections to the prefrontal cortex were severed—as you can imagine, the procedure had widespread cognitive and emotional effects. Electroconvulsive therapy (also called electroshock therapy) began in the late 1930s—this is a treatment for depression, bipolar disorder, and catatonia, and involves inducing seizures in patients with electrical shocks—and it is still used today.

In the 1950s and 1960s a variety of criticisms of psychiatry coalesced into a movement that became known as "anti-psychiatry." This loose movement included famous psychiatrists and philosophers such as Thomas Szasz, R. D. Laing, and Michel Foucault. Conversely, at about the same time as the rise of the anti-psychiatry movement, new psychiatric drugs were introduced that enhanced the credibility of psychiatry—these included the antipsychotic drug chlorpromazine, and the antidepressants iproniazid and imipramine. In subsequent decades more and more psychiatric medications were developed, and now vast numbers of people are prescribed such drugs, to the point where this form of psychiatric treatment has become normalized. In short, beginning in the middle of the twentieth century and onward there are two identifiable opposed positions: antipsychiatry and what we can simply call pro-psychiatry.

We have already seen a hint of an argument for anti-psychiatry, which is based on the gruesome history of psychiatric treatment. Let's call this the *historical* argument for anti-psychiatry. The argument involves uncovering the terrible ways that psychiatry has treated people, and noting that these interventions were ineffective or harmful. Psychiatric diagnosis and intervention has often been used to control deviant behavior rather than to care for or to cure patients.

Indeed, a related argument of anti-psychiatrists is that psychiatry has been used as an instrument of oppression, especially toward people who already suffer from various forms of oppression, including women and minorities. For example, Elizabeth Packard was a woman in the mid-nineteenth century who was unwillingly confined in a hospital for the mentally ill, and her confinement was motivated by her husband, apparently because she did not hold the same fanatic religious beliefs that he did. Her confinement lasted three years. Packard went on to write a number of books about her experience, and she founded the Anti-Insane Asylum Society. Another example of the use of psychiatry for oppression is the alleged disease drapeto-mania, which was said in the nineteenth century to be the cause of slaves fleeing their owners. The first doctor to describe this disease wrote "its diagnostic symptom, the absconding from service, is well known to our planters and overseers" and if a slave owner suspected that one of his slaves had drapetomania, the best preventive measure was "whipping the devil out of them."

Here is a more recent example. In the former Soviet Union political dissidents were diagnosed with "philosophical intoxication" or "sluggish schizophrenia" (symptoms included pessimism and conflict with authorities), and they were involuntarily committed to prison-like hospitals without public trial. Khrushchev, the leader of the Soviet Union in the 1950s, wrote this: "A crime is a deviation from generally recognized standards of behavior frequently caused by mental disorder. . . . Of those who might start calling for opposition to Communism on this basis, we can say that clearly their mental state is not normal." That is, opponents of the political status quo were deemed to have psychiatric diseases and were involuntarily confined and often subject to gruesome treatment.

A crucial premise of the historical argument for anti-psychiatry is that the present is similar to the past in relevant respects. Psychiatry still involves controlling deviant behavior and offers little in the way of real care for patients, is the claim. This, however, is just what pro-psychiatrists would deny. Pro-psychiatrists argue that interventions have become much less invasive and more effective, that involuntary confinement has become rarer and reserved for cases of extreme psychopathy or when a person is a threat to themselves or to others, and psychiatric diagnosis has improved. Anti-psychiatry, in turn, challenges these rejoinders.

Another argument for anti-psychiatry holds that it is not people who are sick with mental disease, it is society. Let's call this the *sick society* argument. The idea is that many features of society—education, employment, government, military, families, police, economy—are dysfunctional. Some people have difficulty coordinating their emotional, cognitive, and behavioral functioning in sick societies, and the sick society identifies such people as having a mental illness. But the sick society argument holds that it is society that is insane, not people. Here is how the twentieth-century psychologist Erich Fromm put it: "An unhealthy society is one which creates mutual hostility, distrust, which transforms man into an instrument of use and exploitation for others, which deprives him of a sense of self, except inasmuch as he submits to others or becomes an automaton." Fromm took inspiration from a quote from the Roman philosopher Seneca: "There exists no more difficult art than living." The idea is that a sick society creates problems in living—in adjusting to the constraints demanded by families, schools, employers, or governments.

Such problems in living can manifest as mental illness, but this illness is not an intrinsic property of a person but rather is a (normal, healthy) response to an unhealthy society. An example of a psychiatric disease that some people cite in this regard is Attention Deficit Hyperactivity Disorder (ADHD): critics claim that ADHD is characterized by normal childhood behavior like moving around and talking with friends, which is exacerbated by the confines of overcrowded classrooms, and does not directly cause difficulty for the child but rather for his schoolteacher (which, of course, tends, indirectly, to cause difficulty for a child).

One might object to the sick society argument by claiming that societies cannot literally be sick. Just think back to chapter 2 and ask how a society could have a condition that satisfied any of the general theories of disease. This is an uncharitable response to the argument, however, because a society does not have to be literally sick to create the conditions under which individuals do not do well in that society.

In chapter 6 we discussed the notion of medicalization. Critics of contemporary psychiatry claim that much of psychiatry involves inappropriate medicalization. An example is depression: some people argue that many cases of depression are in fact normal affective responses to the difficulty of the human condition—sadness after losing one's job, for example, is perfectly normal and not necessarily an indication that one has a disease. It's no wonder so many people appear depressed, goes this argument, because the world can be a depressing place. The worry about medicalization, then, is related to the sick society argument, though they are distinct concerns. Medicalization could occur even in a sane society.

A contemporary argument for anti-psychiatry is more straightforward than the sick society argument, and it is based on the best evidence presently available for many psychiatric interventions. We saw in chapter 10 that an argument for medical nihilism is the small effect sizes of many recent medical interventions. This appears to be an especially salient problem for modern psychiatry. In some meta-analyses that compare antidepressants with placebo, and that have access to both published and unpublished data, the results indicate that antidepressants are hardly better than placebo at alleviating symptoms of depression. Similarly, in the best-designed randomized trials of Ritalin for ADHD, children on Ritalin are no better-off than children on placebo when they are evaluated over the long term. In short, critics claim that although contemporary psychiatric interventions may, on the whole, be less brutal than historical psychiatric interventions, they are not very effective.

So why do so many people think that psychiatric interventions are effective? Present-day anti-psychiatrists point to the actions of pharmaceutical companies as an explanation for widely held misleading beliefs about psychopharmaceuticals. In chapter 8 we studied the role of industry in medical science, how this can lead to conflicts of interest, and ultimately how this can generate publicly available evidence that is unreliable. The argument is that many contemporary psychiatric interventions merely appear effective without in fact being effective, and this is a result of the dubious research practices of companies that manufacture the interventions, the successful marketing tactics employed by these companies, conjoined perhaps with a gullible media and a hopeful populace. Articulated like that, the argument has the flavor of a conspiracy theory. What do you think? Is this argument compelling?

12.4 DELUSIONS AND EXCLUSIONS

Delusions are a strange but fundamental aspect of some psychiatric disorders. One of the goals of philosophy of psychiatry has been to understand what delusions are and to propose theories about their origins. Here is how the *DSM-5* defines them: "Delusions are fixed beliefs that are not amenable to change in light of conflicting evidence. Their content may include a variety of themes (e.g. persecutory, referential, somatic, religious, grandiose). . . . Delusions are deemed bizarre if they are clearly implausible and not understandable to same-culture peers and do not derive from ordinary life experiences." Delusions are a symptom of schizophrenia, dementia, and other serious psychiatric diseases.

The *DSM* definition of delusions is unsatisfactory for a few reasons. One is that most of us hold fixed beliefs that we are unwilling to amend even when conflicting evidence suggests that the belief is false. There is a large amount of psychological research that shows that humans are generally bad at modifying their beliefs even when presented with evidence which disconfirms that belief. Our beliefs are stubborn. As the historian and philosopher of science Thomas Kuhn argued (in his famous book *The Structure of Scientific Revolutions*), even the very best scientists stubbornly stick to scientific beliefs despite disconfirming evidence. Thus, in this respect, a delusion is just like a stubbornly held belief, even a scientific belief. One could respond to this by biting the bullet and agreeing that there is no difference in kind between psychiatric delusions and mere quotidian beliefs that remain unrevised upon receipt of disconfirming evidence. But this seems unfaithful to the extremity of delusions as witnessed from the third-person perspective.

A related issue is how the *DSM* definition of delusion deals with religious beliefs. On the face of it, religious beliefs are "fixed beliefs that are not amenable to change in light of conflicting evidence." So at first pass, religious beliefs are delusions according to this definition. This would be a serious mark against the account, because it would mean that a large proportion of people suffer from the same sort of delusions that psychotic patients suffer from. However, the *DSM* patches this problem by claiming that bizarre delusions must be "clearly implausible" and "not understandable to same-culture peers." This patch, however, only pushes the issue back a level. Religious beliefs, such as the belief in an omnipotent, omniscient, all-loving deity, are in fact clearly implausible to many people.

A defender of this account of delusions could say that religious beliefs are understandable to same-culture peers, and thus do not count as delusions. The problem with this move is that it depends on what one means by same-culture peers. If the boundary of a culture is construed broadly (say, the Euro-American culture), then it follows that many religious beliefs will not be understandable to same-culture peers (for instance, Joe, an atheist, does not understand the religious beliefs of his neighbor, Sam, who is a member of the Church of Latter Day Saints). If, on the other hand, we are permitted to construe the boundary of cultures narrowly (say, the culture of people who are committed to the doctrines of the Church of Latter Day Saints), then religious beliefs clearly will be understandable to same-culture peers, but a different problem arises: a cultural boundary can be drawn so narrowly as to include all and only those people who believe in a particular delusion (say, all those people who believe that the government is controlling their minds with exotic technology), and since these beliefs will clearly be understandable to same-culture peers, no delusional belief can be deemed a delusion.

A response to this issue is just like the response to the first issue. One can say that all beliefs are of a kind: some are relatively well-supported by evidence and reason while others are not. There is a spectrum of justification. Delusions would be on the far end of the unjustified spectrum. Religious beliefs and recalcitrant beliefs would be somewhere more in the middle of the justified spectrum, though still on the empirically unjustified end of the spectrum. Many quotidian beliefs, say, about today's weather or about the name of your mother, would be on the opposite end of the spectrum, as would be many scientific beliefs. This resolves the puzzles above but seems rather unintuitive: delusional beliefs seem of a different kind than, say, poorly substantiated beliefs about the world.

Another interesting dispute regarding delusions is about their genesis. There are two main kinds of theories about the formation of delusions: psychodynamic theories and pathophysiological theories. Psychodynamic theories of delusions claim that delusions arise as a kind of defense mechanism. For example, if I am constantly failing in my job I might develop a delusion that my boss is out to get me.

Pathophysiological theories of delusion claim that delusions arise because of abnormal physiological functioning—usually abnormal cognitive functioning that results from neurological damage.

To distinguish these types of theories, consider the "Capgras delusion," which is a type of delusion in which a person believes that a partner, family member, or friend has been replaced by a seemingly identical imposter. A psychodynamic explanation of Capgras delusion would attempt to explain a token instance of the delusion by the functional role the delusion plays for a patient. For example, a daughter who is sexually abused by her father might suffer from the delusion that her father has been replaced by a stranger, and it is the stranger who hurts her so terribly. Conversely, a pathophysiological explanation of Capgras delusion would appeal to whatever is known about the cognitive or neuroscientific basis of the delusion, such as memory problems and abnormalities in the neuronal activity of the frontal lobe.

Let's turn to a different but equally perplexing issue. We saw in chapter 6 and §12.2 that some critics of psychiatry claim that many alleged cases of psychiatric disease are just normal responses to life's difficulties. The idea is that, sometimes, particular difficult aspects of a person's life can explain the presence of symptoms better than the postulation that this person has a disease. For example, if I am especially jittery and fidgety, this is because I drink too much coffee, and not because I have an anxiety disorder.

The previous edition of the *DSM*, the *DSM-IV*, incorporated such thinking into its definition of depression, by claiming that if a person satisfied the diagnostic criteria for depression then that person should be diagnosed with depression *unless* that person was bereaving the death of a loved one. The idea was this: if a person was bereaving, then they might satisfy the diagnostic criteria of depression but not in fact have depression, because, after all, it is normal to experience some of those symptoms after the death of a loved one. This was called the "bereavement exclusion criterion" for depression. In principle there could be many such exclusion criteria, such as the loss of one's job (since that could also cause symptoms of depression), and there are many more technical exclusion criteria for most psychiatric disorders, but bereavement was the most prominent example of an exclusion criterion for a psychiatric diagnosis based on particular difficult aspects of a person's life.

When the *DSM-5* was published (in 2013), one of the most controversial changes from the previous edition was the elimination of the bereavement exclusion criterion for depression. Now, if a person satisfies the diagnostic criteria for depression, and their spouse died three weeks ago, that person can be diagnosed with depression. Critics of the change argue that this amounts to medicalizing normal but difficult aspects of life, such as grief caused by death of a spouse. Indeed, the charge of psychiatric medicalization is akin to claiming that psychiatry should employ far more such exclusion criteria. On the other hand, proponents of the change argue that bereavement does not somehow "immunize" a person against depression; on the contrary, tragic life events like the death of a loved one can cause depression. Moreover, there is something odd about excluding a person from a diagnosis on the grounds that an event in that person's life can explain the presence of would-be symptoms.

To take an extreme example, suppose I take a risk while riding my bicycle without a helmet, and I get into an accident and fracture my skull. It would be strange to say that I do not have a head injury, on the grounds that my would-be symptoms can be explained by the fact that I took a risk while riding my bicycle and got into an accident. The crucial premise of the pro-exclusion criteria camp seems to be that would-be symptoms should be explained by *either* a difficult life event *or* the presence of a disease; the rejoinder is that this is a false dichotomy, precisely because a difficult life event can precipitate the presence of a disease. Nevertheless, in psychiatry there is something compelling about the intuition that many sets of would-be symptoms are not brought about by the presence of a disease but rather are normal responses to the difficulties of life.

FURTHER READING

Psychiatric nosology: Murphy (2006), Tabb (2015), Tsou (2011), Murphy (2010)

Anti-psychiatry: Foucault (1965 [1961])
Delusions: Bortolotti (2009), Parrott (2016)

DISCUSSION QUESTIONS

1. How should psychiatry construct its disease categories?
2. When it comes to defining and assessing the effectiveness of medical interventions, should psychiatry be held to the same standards as other branches of medicine?
3. Should diseases like depression have diagnostic exclusion criteria, such as bereavement due to loss of a family member or stress due to loss of a job?
4. Is the anti-psychiatry movement relevant to contemporary psychiatry?

13.1 SUMMARY

There are many kinds of policies that pertain to medicine, including political policies, some of which are concerned with the form that a national healthcare system takes; ethical policies, which are concerned with questions such as the permissibility of euthanasia; or economic policies, including which sorts of interventions a healthcare system should pay for. Many such policies are shot through with philosophical concerns. Given the vast range of such policies, we can study only a few domains in which philosophical problems permeate policy deliberations pertinent to medicine. This chapter addresses several policy questions that are relevant to medical research (and not, say, medical treatment, or the social structure of medical systems).

Before any research is actually performed, scientists must determine what problems to study. In science generally there are two very broad motivations to pursue a particular research question: intellectual curiosity and practical importance. Because medicine is by its nature a practical activity, the motivation of practical importance is dominant. But what makes a research question important? And who should decide whether or not a research question is important?

Another important philosophical question pertinent to policy about medical science is whether or not the products of medical research should be protected by intellectual property laws. Many discoveries in science, including medical science, are protected by such laws, which grant to the discoverer control over the manufacture and sale of that which is discovered (such as a new drug). Intellectual property laws are fully entrenched in our society. Recently, however, these laws have been criticized, especially in the domain of medicine. We study the main arguments that have been raised to justify intellectual property laws, and then assess their plausibility when applied to medical science.

In this chapter we'll also assess philosophical questions pertaining to regulatory policy. In order for a new medical intervention to be made available to patients, it must be approved by the appropriate regulatory agency. In the United States the regulatory agency that approves new drugs is the Food and Drug Administration (FDA); in Europe it is the European Medicines Agency (EMA). The main methodological standards of these two regulators are similar, but in this chapter we examine the FDA standard as a focus for evaluation. Some critics of current drug regulation claim that regulators are too strict in their regulation, while other critics claim that regulators are not strict enough. We examine the arguments on both sides.

13.2 RESEARCH PRIORITIES

Vast resources are devoted to medical research. But some argue that these resources are not used fairly and efficiently. Both radical and moderate solutions have been proposed to address this maldistribution of resources.

Most clinical research today is funded by private companies. These companies tend to pursue research projects that will lead to profitable products. Usually such products are medical interventions for diseases that more often affect people in the West, such as heart disease and depression, rather than diseases that more often affect people in poor countries, such as malaria. This is called the "10/90 gap": 10% of the world's medical research resources are used to study health problems of 90% of the world's population (and this 90% is the world's poorest). To put this differently, 90% of the world's medical research resources are used to study diseases that affect 10% of the world's population.

Here's a specific example of how the present system of medical research does not distribute its research resources very well: there has been little research on new antibiotics in recent years because a new antibiotic would not be prescribed very often. Due to the development of antibiotic-resistant bacteria we desperately need new antibiotics, but any new addition to the arsenal of antibiotics would be reserved for the most extreme cases of infections with bacteria that are resistant to all previous antibiotics (since new antibiotics would not be prescribed very often, private companies have little incentive to develop them). Also, patients are on antibiotics for only a few days or weeks at a time, whereas patients have to take other kinds of drugs (such as statins, antidepressants, or birth control pills) for months or years. So, there is little incentive for pharmaceutical companies to research new antibiotics, despite the fact that it is very important for us to develop new antibiotics.

Thus we are in a situation in which a great amount of medical research is taking place, but the research resources are not properly distributed. What should be done about this? This is a political question, and thus a compelling answer will involve political theory. Two main competing views regarding the distribution of research resources are libertarianism and socialism. Libertarianism holds that people and companies should be free to focus their research resources however they wish. Socialism holds that research resources should be controlled by central government authorities.

Let's consider the arguments in favor of libertarianism about the medical research agenda. There are two main arguments for this position. One is derivative on libertarianism more generally: libertarians believe that people should be free to do what they want as long as their actions do not hurt others. This applies to scientific research. If a scientist wants to research x, and researching x does not harm others, then that scientist should be free to research x. People and companies should be free to use their resources as they wish, goes this argument, and so as long as the resources belong to the scientist (or her employer), that scientist should be free to research x. Suppose a company has, say, one billion dollars, and its management decides to investigate a new drug for treating baldness—on what grounds could one keep them from doing this? A problem with this argument is that research resources are finite, and a particular distribution of finite resources can in fact harm people. To take an example from above, the 10/90 gap harms people who suffer from under-investigated diseases. Thus, goes this rejoinder, a free choice to dedicate research resources to a particular problem (say, baldness), can in fact have the consequence that people with other medical problems (say, malaria) are harmed.

The other main argument for libertarianism about the medical research agenda is based on the idea that the very nature of science requires a commitment to unfettered free inquiry. Libertarians cite examples such as the Lysenko affair to illustrate this point. Lysenko was a Soviet agricultural scientist who was very popular with the Soviet Communist Party, and who advocated a theory of evolution based on Lamarckian principles (this was the idea of "inheritance of acquired characteristics"). Thousands of scientists who doubted Lysenko were fired, executed, or sent to labor camps. This was a great loss, of course, and a major setback for science—beyond the tragic loss of these scientists, science was set back because of the political constraints placed on the scientific research agenda. An explicit premise of this argument is that truth can be most readily obtained when the research agenda is uncontrolled. Are you convinced by this premise? An implicit premise of this argument is that truth is the ambition of science. This is often the case for much of science. However, when applied to medical science, practical concerns (like caring for patients or curing diseases) are more pressing than intellectual concerns. It is far from clear that the goal of satisfying such practical concerns can most readily be obtained when the medical research agenda is uncontrolled.

Now let's consider the arguments in favor of socialism about the medical research agenda. Again, there are two main arguments in favor of this position. The first follows on from the consideration we just assessed about the efficiency of medical science to achieve its ambition of satisfying the practical concerns of care and cure. Proponents of socialized medical research argue that medicine would be better able to care for patients and cure diseases if the medical research agenda were guided by democratic deliberation rather than private whim. Socialists sometimes cite the example of *me-too drugs* as an illustration of this point. Me-too drugs are drugs that are very similar to preexisting drugs already on the market, such as new types of selective serotonin reuptake inhibitors for depression. They are called "me-too drugs" because if one company is making great profit by selling a drug of type x, then a competitor company will say "me-too" and introduce its own new drug of type x in an attempt to earn some of that profit. One estimate is that me-too drugs make up about 75% of new drugs. The problem is that me-too drugs do not bring much additional benefit for patients. Once we have a drug of type x, having a second drug of type x does not much enhance medicine's capacity to care and cure.

A similar illustration of the inefficiency of libertarian distribution of medical research resources is based on "neglected tropical diseases." This term applies to diseases that tend to affect poor people disproportionately more than wealthy people, and they tend to be infectious diseases—tropical infectious diseases cause a profound amount of suffering and receive very little attention by medical science (hence the term neglected tropical diseases). The proportion of medical research resources that neglected tropical diseases have received relative to the suffering these diseases cause is far, far less than that received by diseases that tend to affect wealthy countries, such as chronic diseases like heart disease, cancer, and diabetes. Even just a small redistribution of research resources away from these chronic diseases and toward neglected tropical diseases could greatly enhance the capacity of medicine to care and cure, goes this socialist argument from efficiency (which is ultimately based on consequentialism).

The second argument for socialism about the distribution of medical research resources is based on an analogy with socialism about the distribution of medical care. Unlike the first argument, which was motivated by a consideration of efficiency, this argument is motivated by a consideration of fairness. Here's the idea: most of us believe that medical *delivery* should be socialized. The vast majority of countries have socialized systems of healthcare delivery, on the grounds of fairness (it strikes most people as grossly unfair that some people should be denied treatment simply because they cannot afford private healthcare or health insurance). The argument from analogy is this: since medical delivery is socialized, medical research should also be socialized. If one thinks that medical treatment ought not be part of the free market, then one should also think that medical research ought not be part of the free market, goes this argument. An argument from analogy is only as good as the tightness of the analogy. What do you make of this analogy?

A notion developed by Philip Kitcher called *well-ordered science* can be applied to this debate between socialism and libertarianism regarding medical research resources. Science is well-ordered, according to Kitcher, only if it is directed in ways that promote common goals. Common goals are those that are endorsed in democratic deliberation among well-informed participants, who have in mind the ends of others. One common goal that such deliberators would share is the scientific study of problems of significance, where these satisfy basic human curiosity or have practical importance. Science is well ordered if it pursues these problems of significance. Moreover, for science to be well ordered, it has to distribute its research resources proportionate to the relative significance of the many problems it addresses. Phenomena such as the 10/90 gap and neglected tropical diseases indicate that medical science is not presently well-ordered.

13.3 INTELLECTUAL PROPERTY

Intellectual property rights are a cluster of laws that grant ownership privileges to inventors. In medical science the most common type of intellectual property right is a patent. A patent is a set of rights granted to an inventor by a state in exchange for making details of the invention public. The rights granted to an inventor by a patent typically include a temporary monopoly on producing and selling the invented product. Patents prohibit other people (or companies) from making or selling the product, and in some countries this prohibition usually lasts for twenty years from the time a patent is granted.

The very first intellectual property law is the Statute of Anne, passed by the parliament of Great Britain in 1710. Here is the preamble to the law:

"Whereas printers, booksellers, and other persons, have of late frequently taken the liberty of printing, reprinting, and publishing, or causing to be printed, reprinted, and published, books and other writings, without the consent of the authors or proprietors of such books and writings, to their very great detriment, and too often to the ruin of them and their families: for preventing therefore such practices for the future, and for the encouragement of learned men to compose and write useful books. . . ." This law, in other words, was motivated by the desire to protect writers and to incentivize the creation of new written work. Intellectual property laws have expanded

to cover all sorts of inventions, including technical inventions resulting from scientific research.

In medical science, clinical research on an experimental intervention usually begins after the intervention has been patented. We saw
in chapter 7 that in order to get regulatory approval a new pharmaceutical must first be tested in animals, then in phase 1 trials, then in
phase 2 trials, and finally in multiple phase 3 trials (we study this in a
bit more detail in the next section, §13.4). This entire process can take
around ten years. So companies typically have around ten years left
on the patent of a new intervention once that intervention has been
granted regulatory approval.

There are several different kinds of arguments that purport to justify the granting of intellectual property rights. One is based on the labor that an inventor uses in creating a novel product: the idea is that
when one uses one's labor to modify or create an object, one thereby
gains property rights over that object, and this holds for intellectual
objects. This justification of intellectual property was developed by
the seventeenth century philosopher John Locke. The second (though
similar) kind of argument for intellectual property rights is based
on the idea that the creation of both material and intellectual products is the result of an individual's creativity, and thus is an expression of one's personality; since it is intuitive to think that one should
have some control over the manifestations of our personalities, one
should be granted property rights over those manifestations. This
justification of intellectual property is based on the work of Hegel,
who held that one should be entitled to have control over the material
and intellectual expressions of one's talents and personality.

The main problem for both of these arguments is that it is mysterious how one's labor or personality can be "mixed" with material or
intellectual objects such that one thereby gains property rights over
those objects. This is especially problematic in medical science, in
which there is little personality involved in the research, and the relevant labor is distributed over many scientists. As we saw in chapter 8, one of the features that helps science to achieve some degree
of objectivity is its social structure, involving many people in various
roles, and the skills associated with these roles are developed and

maintained over time in a complex social nexus (and thus it is not the case that one can simply "own" one's scientific skills and talents, as one owns a pair of shoes).

The third main argument that has been offered to justify intellectual property, and the one that most people find compelling at least in the context of scientific research, is consequentialist. This argument holds that intellectual property rights incentivize research and development of innovative products. In medical science such products are interventions that are supposed to improve our health. Thus, goes this reasoning, the granting of intellectual property rights can have significant beneficial consequences, such as improving our health. Since those consequences are good, goes this argument, we should grant intellectual property rights.

Critics of the practice of granting intellectual property rights note that the above utilitarian argument has an empirical premise that is, at least in the domain of medical science, false. Intellectual property rights in medicine do not always incentivize research and development of innovative health-improving products. Indeed, some critics claim that intellectual property rights incentivize research and development of me-too drugs, which we learned about in the previous section, §13.2. Moreover, the temporary monopoly guaranteed by patents entails that companies can charge whatever they want for important medications, and this can hurt healthcare systems and ultimately lead to less access to medicine. This is another way in which the granting of intellectual property rights in medicine can lead to harmful consequences.

A related problem is that since the incentive to develop new drugs is based on financial profit from selling drugs under patent, many diseases are neglected. This includes rare diseases and diseases that primarily affect people in poor countries, such as tropical diseases like malaria. Companies have little incentive to research new drugs for diseases that occur very rarely because they can sell only a small number of treatments for those diseases. Companies have little incentive to research new drugs for diseases that affect poor countries because they can charge only a little amount per treatment. Similarly, companies have little incentive to research new antibiotics—

given the development of antibiotic resistance in bacteria, a new antibiotic would be rarely used and instead would be saved for patients with infections that are resistant to all other preexisting antibiotics. Unfortunately, as we saw in §13.2, diseases that affect poor countries and infectious diseases for which we could use new antibiotics are among the most harmful diseases, and so research and development of new treatments for these diseases would be valuable, yet the patent system disincentivizes such research. This is a challenge to the consequentialist justification of granting intellectual property rights in medical science, since the financial incentives that arise due to the granting of intellectual property rights in fact bring about these very negative consequences.

Finally, critics of intellectual property in medicine note that important scientific breakthroughs generally occur in the absence of intellectual property rights. This is the case for science at large and for medicine in particular. Consider general scientific advances, such as Galileo's astronomical observations that lent support to the sun-centered model of the solar system, Darwin's discovery of evolution by natural selection, or Einstein's theory of relativity. These scientific breakthroughs were not incentivized by the financial gain to be had by intellectual property rights. This is also the case for the great medical breakthroughs in history, such as the discovery of x-rays, the discovery of insulin as a cure for diabetes, or the development of the polio vaccine.

For the above reasons, some critics claim that patents should be eliminated from medical research. A counter-argument to this proposal is that in the absence of the potential for financial profit thanks to patents, companies would have little incentive to research and develop new medical interventions. This counter-argument is rather question-begging, since we have already seen that this incentive is not necessary for important medical breakthroughs. Nevertheless, to mitigate this potential worry, some critics opt for complementary or more modest policies. For instance, some critics hold that patents should not be immediately eliminated, but rather the duration of patent protection should gradually be decreased and the effects of this should be carefully observed. Others hold that patents should be immediately eliminated, but to guarantee that new medical interventions continue to be researched and developed, such scientific activity should become the responsibility of the state.

A more modest proposal is to more rigorously enforce preexisting patent rules. In most jurisdictions, to get a patent on an invention, the invention must meet certain requirements: in the US, to be patentable inventions must be novel, useful, and non-obvious. To respond to the problem of me-too drugs, for instance, patent offices could more strictly uphold these requirements—me-too drugs are not very novel, useful, or non-obvious. Another modest proposal is to keep the patent system but provide other ways of incentivizing diverse biomedical research, such as prizes and government-funded awards. This proposal could mitigate the problem of certain diseases being neglected by current medical science.

13.4 STANDARDS FOR REGULATION

Regulatory agencies, such as the Food and Drug Administration (FDA) in the United States or the European Medicines Agency (EMA) in Europe, are responsible for ensuring that drugs are safe and effective. In order to market, sell, or prescribe a drug, that drug must be approved by such regulatory agencies. Experimental drugs must meet certain standards in order to be approved. We will focus here on the current FDA standard. Some commentators claim that this standard is fine, allowing useful drugs to be available to patients while keeping most harmful drugs off the market. Other commentators claim that this standard is bad because it is too cumbersome—it keeps useful drugs off the market, and it increases the cost of developing drugs and so increases cost to patients, and thus the FDA is "overregulating." Still other commentators claim that the regulatory standard is bad because it is too loose—it allows unsafe or ineffective drugs on the market and thus the regulatory agency is "underregulating." Which is the right view?

First, let's get clear on the regulatory standard. (We are focusing here on the evidential standards and not on other standards that pertain to the regulation of medical interventions, such as production standards.) In most cases, the standard for new drug approval is that there must be two phase 3 randomized trials that show that the new drug is more effective than placebo, and these findings must be statistically significant. These are called "positive" trials. For a reminder of what phase 3 trials are, see chapter 7, and for a reminder of what statistical significance means, see chapter 9. There are exceptions to this standard—for example, sometimes only one phase 3 trial is required, and sometimes an intervention is approved with no randomized trial at all—but for most interventions the standard applies.

Regulators must make a judgment about the effectiveness and safety of a new medical intervention, on the basis of the evidence that is submitted to them. That is, regulators must make a causal inference, and there are two basic errors regulators can commit: they can approve a drug as being relatively safe and effective when it in fact is not, or they can reject a drug as not being relatively safe and effective when it in fact is. The former error (mistaken drug approval) harms patients by allowing ineffective and unsafe drugs on the market, and the latter error (mistaken drug rejection) harms patients by prohibiting effective and safe drugs and can harm the financial interests of the companies that make the drug.

One might think that the current regulatory standard is fine because of the rigor and control that go into phase 3 randomized trials. A phase 3 trial involves many subjects and is typically very expensive and involves many methodological safeguards (chapter 7). To require two positive trials is sufficient to guarantee that most approved drugs are safe and effective, according to defenders of the standard. Since the positive finding must occur in not just one but two trials, this ensures that a single positive finding was not just a chancy event or the result of a single biased trial. A problem with this argument is that trials can be biased in numerous ways, which entails that a positive finding might be due to the bias rather than the real effectiveness of a drug. Multiple trials can be biased in the same way, which renders the confirmatory power of multiple positive trials moot. For example, in §8.2 we learned about publication bias, which saps the confirmatory power of multiple positive trials that suggest a drug is effective, since we know that negative trials are withheld from publication.

Another argument that suggests that the current standard is good is that few drugs are removed from the market once a drug is approved. The idea is that if the regulatory standard were not good, then, after drugs had been approved, many would be subsequently withdrawn from the market once their true lack of safety or effectiveness were discovered. This argument is unsound, because the premise—that regulators would withdraw drugs that are found to be unsafe or ineffective—is false.

There are many examples of ineffective and unsafe drugs being left on the market. Some people argue that once the FDA has approved a drug it has a disincentive to apply further regulatory action on that drug, out of fear of admitting a mistake. Moreover, once a drug is approved, the manufacturer of the drug has little incentive to fund further research on its safety and effectiveness. So the majority of new (post–regulatory approval) evidence about a drug comes from clinical use of the drug, but such information is generated in an uncontrolled, unblinded, non-experimental context: basically, such evidence is merely a collection of anecdotes from patients and physicians. As we saw in chapter 7, there are numerous forms of bias associated with such evidence, which is precisely why medical science denigrates such evidence in favor of carefully controlled studies.

Here is another way to put the problem with the above argument. Let's distinguish between two standards a drug can be held to: the current regulatory standard and what we can call the "clinical performance standard." The argument goes like this: the regulatory standard is vindicated because few drugs that satisfy the regulatory standard do not also satisfy the clinical performance standard. The problem is that we do not in fact have good evidence that many drugs satisfy the clinical performance standard. Indeed, as suggested in §10.3, the "medical nihilism" thesis holds that there are plenty of medical interventions that are not very safe and effective. Moreover, the argument is an attempt to vindicate one epistemic standard (namely, the current regulatory standard) by appeal to another epistemic standard (namely, the clinical performance standard), but for the causal inferences in question (namely, assessing the safety and effectiveness of new medical interventions) the former standard is more reliable than the latter standard. So the reliability of the current regulatory

standard cannot be established by appealing to the clinical performance standard.

Some critics of the current regulatory standard claim that it is excessively stringent. To require two positive trials is unnecessary to guarantee that most approved drugs are safe and effective, according to such
critics. The idea is that regulatory agencies currently overregulate. If a
single positive trial suggests that a new drug is safe and effective, then
requiring a second trial simply adds expense and delays the introduction of the drug, thereby harming both the manufacturer of the drug and
patients who could benefit from the drug. We saw above, in the discussion of intellectual property, that new drugs are protected by patent for
twenty years, during which all of the clinical research for its regulatory
approval must occur, and so the regulatory standard requiring multiple phase 3 trials cuts into the amount of time a new drug is both mar-
ketable and protected by patent. So, the regulatory standard cuts into
the profitability of a new drug and thus cuts into the financial incentive
for developing new drugs. Easing the regulatory standard, on this line
of thinking, would permit medical interventions to be made available
to patients more quickly, and the interventions would ultimately be
cheaper. A premise of this line of reasoning, which seems to be widely
held, is that regulation mitigates scientific and medical progress. In response, you might argue that higher regulatory standards would force
companies to develop truly safe and effective interventions because if
they didn't then they would be less competitive than other companies.

Other critics of the current regulatory standard claim that the standard is not stringent enough. Critics who charge regulators with underregulation note several problems with the current regulatory standard.
Critics claim that it is too easy to satisfy, it is epistemologically flawed,
and it thereby permits the approval of unsafe or ineffective drugs.
One problem is that the standard does not take into account how
many trials have been performed on a new drug: there might be two
positive trials but ten negative trials. The negative trials may or may
not have been published. As we saw in chapter 8, publication bias
is a serious problem in medical research, and the two-positive-trial
standard inherits the problem of publication bias. Another problem
with the standard is that it is based on frequentist statistics. We learned

in chapter 9 that frequentist statistical tests can lead to false positive inferences. The current regulatory standard is explicitly committed to inferring that a drug is safe and effective if trials generate data that, when analyzed with frequentist statistical tests, give low p-values for the respective null hypotheses. This standard commits both types of frequentist inference fallacies discussed in chapter 9 (the "reject ~H" fallacy and the "accept H" fallacy). A related problem is that a statistically significant result in a trial might be due to the new drug having a real but very small beneficial effect, so small that it is clinically insignificant. Finally, as we learned in chapter 9, extrapolating from trials to the real world population of patients is not straightforward, yet the FDA standard assumes that if a drug is found to be safe and effective in a trial population then we can infer that it will be safe and effective in the real world population of patients.

So there are arguments to support the regulatory status quo, arguments to support the view that regulators are overregulating new drugs, and arguments to support the view that regulators are underregulating new drugs. Which view do you find most believable?

One final noteworthy issue about the debate between those who charge regulators with underregulation versus those who charge regulators with overregulation is that non-epistemic values have an influence in the debate. In chapter 8 we studied the argument from inductive risk, which challenges the value-free ideal of science. This argument is pertinent to regulation. If regulators err on the side of overregulation, then they will reject too many drugs (or at least slow down the approval process), which thereby denies patients drugs and hurts the manufacturers. If, on the other hand, regulators err on the side of underregulation, then they will approve too many mediocre drugs, which will harm patients. Which of these sets of harms is more important? To answer that requires appealing to non-epistemic values, like social, political, economic, or ethical values.

FURTHER READING

Standards for regulation: Stegenga (2017), Teira (2017)
Intellectual property: Brown (2008), Biddle (2014)
Research priorities: Kitcher (2001), Brown (2008)

1. Should the results of medical science be protected by intellectual property laws? Why or why not?
2. Who should set the biomedical research agenda? How should it be set?
3. If you could rewrite the evidential standards for drug regulation, what evidence would you require for a new drug to be approved?
4. Do patents incentivize innovative medical research?

14 : PUBLIC HEALTH

Most of medicine is concerned with the health of individuals, the diseases that individuals can get, and interventions that individuals can use. Public health, however, is different. Public health is a branch of medicine that is concerned with the health of populations, the population-level causes of disease, and interventions that are administered to populations to improve health.

The discipline of "social epidemiology" or "social medicine" investigates "social" factors, or features of society, that influence health and disease. For example, social epidemiologists study the influence of poverty on rates of obesity. An influential though controversial thesis in social epidemiology is that such social factors have been the dominant cause of the improvements to health that industrial societies have witnessed over the past couple of centuries. In other words, these improvements in health—such as the decrease in childhood mortality, increase in lifespan, and lower rates of mortal infectious diseases—are less the result of improvements in medical interventions (like new drugs) and more the result of public health measures (such as access to clean drinking water) and improvements in social conditions (such as greater socioeconomic equality and prosperity). We start this chapter by assessing this thesis.

A major endeavor of public health is known as "preventive medicine." The basic idea of preventive medicine is simple: we ought to strive toward avoiding the development of diseases in the first place, rather than waiting until a disease has appeared and only then trying to intervene upon it. Rather than fight fires, we should strive to avoid fires. The idea hardly seems controversial. However, preventive medicine pushes the boundary of the domain of medicine. For example, eating well is a preventive means to avoid clogged arteries, but is nutritional guidance on eating well properly part of medicine? Wearing a seatbelt is a preventive means to avoid an injury in a car crash, but are seatbelts and seatbelt laws part of medicine? This is another point of dispute between reductionists and holists (chapter 5).

One puzzle about preventive medicine is that the vast majority of people who use preventive interventions do not benefit from them. We saw this issue arise with respect to screening, which is essentially a preventive practice (chapter 11). And yet such interventions can bring about a great deal of benefit, such as saving many lives. Some people call this a paradox. We'll see why, and offer a straightforward resolution of the paradox.

Health inequalities are a deeply disturbing fact of modern life. For instance, wealthy people in the southeast of England live, on average, over eight years longer than poor people in the north of England. Facts like this strike many people as unjust. We end this chapter by investigating some of the nuances of health inequalities.

14.2 SOCIAL EPIDEMIOLOGY

The study of frequencies, distributions, and causes of diseases occurs in the domain of medicine called *epidemiology*. A particular subdiscipline is "social epidemiology," which studies the influence of social factors on disease.

Consider a famous example of social epidemiology. The Whitehall Study was a famous epidemiological investigation into the social determinants of health. This study looked at thousands of British civil servants ("Whitehall" refers to the central British government administration), and found a strong correlation between the "grade" (or rank) of the civil servants and the frequency of mortality caused by a variety of diseases. Lower rank was associated with obesity, smoking, lower levels of physical activity, and higher blood pressure, yet even after controlling for all of these factors, lower grade civil servants had higher rates of death by cardiovascular disease. This study was led by the well-known epidemiologist Michael Marmot. Marmot offered as an explanation for this correlation between social rank and health the mediating role of stress: the hypothesis is that lower-ranking civil servants have less control over their work life and thus experience more stress, and stress is a cause of poor health outcomes.

Such work is concerned with discovering the "social determinants of health"—the social and economic factors that cause disparities in health outcomes. Social determinants of health are causes that influence one's health that are extrinsic to an individual person's physiology and are structural features of one's social context. Other empirical studies suggest that, in addition to stress and social rank, social factors that can negatively impact one's health include social isolation, unemployment, food insecurity, and income distribution. These factors are not independent of each other, of course—for example, unemployment is correlated with poverty, social isolation, and food insecurity.

Another famous contribution to social epidemiology used historical records to study the causes of changing diseases frequencies over time: in chapter 4 we learned about the "McKeown thesis," developed by the physician and historian of medicine Thomas McKeown in the 1970s. McKeown argued that the growth in populations since the industrial revolution was fuelled by a decline in mortality caused by improved standards of living (particularly improved nutrition), and that innovations in medical interventions played little role in the decline of mortality. The idea is that the industrial revolution generated a degree of economic prosperity for many people and contributed to the development of a large middle class. This meant that many more people than before were able to satisfy basic nutritional needs, which itself improved people's health. One of McKeown's examples is the decline in tuberculosis rates. You might think that tuberculosis rates decreased after the introduction of antibiotics, but McKeown noted that tuberculosis rates began falling long before that. These developments led to a decline in mortality rates and a concomitant increase in average lifespan.

The thesis that medical interventions had less to do with the increase in lifespan than did socioeconomic factors lends some support to the "medical nihilism" thesis, discussed in chapter 10. That's because one objection to medical nihilism is the fact that our average health has improved so much over the past two centuries. Even just in the past few decades the average lifespan has been increasing. One possible explanation for this is the development of great medical interventions. However, if the McKeown thesis is correct, then that alleged explanation is far less compelling.

The McKeown thesis has been challenged by critics. For example, the Cambridge Group for the History of Population and Social Structure examined parish registers beginning from the sixteenth century onward, to conclude that population increase was largely due to an increase in fertility. Some critics have argued that McKeown overstated his case, because sanitation and other public health initiatives were important to lowering mortality. Access to clean drinking water, for example, or hygienic sewage systems, evidently contributed to public health.

Nevertheless, such criticisms of the McKeown thesis amount to pointing out other public health measures that contributed to overall improvements in health. That is, such criticisms hold that it was not *simply* the improvement in greater socioeconomic equality that led to improvements in nutrition and thereby improvements in health; there were other improvements to social determinants of health that were responsible for such improvements in health. Notice, though, how much this objection concedes. This response to the McKeown thesis basically augments the social determinants of health that McKeown noted with other social determinants of health; the rejoinder doesn't show that mainstream medical interventions such as pharmaceuticals also played an important role in the improvement of health in the past two centuries. The question remains: Were medical interventions a significant cause of the increase in health witnessed in the past couple of centuries?

This general question has much more concrete and specific manifestations in contemporary public health policy. Policy-makers must determine which medical interventions to pay for. Organizations like the National Institute for Health and Care Excellence (NICE), which is a public institution in the United Kingdom involved in what is called "health technology assessment," are responsible for such decisions. To do so, such organizations need an estimate of how much benefit different interventions will bring, at a population level.

One important measure that organizations such as NICE use is the "quality-adjusted life year," or QALY. This measure combines quantified information about how much gain in life expectancy a medical intervention brings with information about the quality of that added time to life. Then, the QALY of various interventions is compared with their cost, and a measure called the *incremental cost-effectiveness ratio* (ICER) of each medical intervention is calculated. Basically, policy-makers need to decide how much they are willing to pay for an increase of one QALY. Today the ICER threshold for NICE is about £20,000-£30,000/QALY. If a new medical intervention has, say, an ICER value of £12,000, it will be recommended for purchase.

Consider this example. The drug trastuzumab emtansine (Kadcyla) is used for late-stage terminal breast cancer, and it was approved by the FDA in 2013 because it appears to extend the lives of patients with late-stage breast cancer from about 25 months to about 31 months. However, FDA approval only means that the drug can be sold to pa-tients, and it does not mean that insurance companies or national healthcare plans will pay for it. Because the original estimate cost of the treatment was £166,000 per QALY, NICE recommended against its use by the United Kingdom National Health Service (later the UK struck a deal with the manufacturer of the drug, Roche, which brought the price of the drug more in line with UK guidelines).

14.3 PREVENTIVE MEDICINE

Preventive medicine, as its name suggests, is concerned with the pre-vention of disease rather than the treatment of disease. It's a simple and compelling idea. Take an extreme example: we'd be far better off avoiding a broken leg than treating a broken leg. But in this simple idea lurks several puzzles.

The epidemiologist Geoffrey Rose described what he called the "prevention paradox." This is a phenomenon in which a large num-ber of people who have a small risk for a particular disease may gen-erate more cases of the disease than a small number of people who have a larger risk for that disease. It follows that if policy-makers want to reduce the number of cases of that disease, they might be better off using interventions that focus on people at low risk of the disease. This in turn entails that most people who are exposed to the intervention will not benefit from the intervention (since they were at low risk of the disease, they most likely would not have developed the disease in any case).

Let's consider a concrete example. Suppose a population is composed of two subpopulations of people at two different risk levels for disease d: a high-risk population (H) that has a 0.2 probability of developing d, and a low-risk population (L) that has a 0.01 probability of developing d. There are 1000 people in H and 1,000,000 in L. Suppose a drug has a relative risk reduction for d of 30%. (Exercise for the reader: What is the risk difference of the drug in H and in L? See §8.4.) A policy-maker must decide to give the drug to members of either H or L, but not both. If policy-makers give the drug to H, the number of people who will develop d will go from 200 (0.2 × 1000) to 140 (30% reduction of 200), and so 60 cases of d will be avoided. On the other hand, if policy-makers give the drug to L, the number of people who will develop d will go from 10,000 (0.01 × 1,000,000) to 7000 (30% reduction of 10,000), and so 3000 cases of d will be avoided. Thus, much more benefit is gained by employing the preventive medical intervention for the low-risk group than the high-risk group.

We saw in chapter 11 that screening programs are like this. Consider another example: statins. Statins are used to lower cholesterol levels, which in turn is meant to lower the risk of heart attacks, and thus statins are a preventive medical intervention. In most demographic groups (which happen to be at low risk of heart attacks), physicians would have to give about one hundred people statins for several years in order to avoid a single heart attack. So, if the benefit of statins is characterized as the actual avoidance of a heart attack, the vast majority of people who use the medical intervention do not benefit from it. And yet, if the intervention were promoted by a public health campaign that led to ten million people consuming statins, then 100,000 heart attacks would be avoided. So the apparent paradox is that no typical individual can expect to benefit from statins, but at the population level many people will benefit.

On the other hand, if the benefit of a preventive medical intervention is characterized as the lowering of one's risk, then (presuming that statins lower everyone's risk of heart attacks by a tiny amount), everyone who takes a statin benefits, if only very slightly. Thus the paradox disappears. The paradox could reappear on this characterization of benefit if consuming an intervention came along with some harm, even if very minor, such as the costs of the intervention, the annoyance of consuming the intervention, and its harmful side effects. Statins, like all drugs, have some financial cost, and statins also have some side effects, and it could be the case that for a particular individual, these costs and harms do not outweigh the benefit of the small lowered risk of a heart attack. Thus, again, in this scenario the average individual would not benefit from the preventive intervention, despite the fact that a great benefit seemingly arises at the population level.

This is only apparently paradoxical, however. If it is in fact the case that, on average, at the individual level the small costs of the intervention outweigh the small benefits of the intervention, then at the population level those small costs sum just as the small benefits sum. And so, if this were the case, then even if statins, as a preventive intervention, could cause a reduction of 100,000 heart attacks when used by ten million people, the population-level costs would still outweigh this population-level benefit.

Preventive medicine used to refer to various lifestyle behaviors that were good for one's health, such as proper diet and regular exercise, and visiting one's doctor regularly for routine checkups. These are undoubtedly good practices and surely benefit many people's health. But preventive medicine has developed into a set of practices that appears very similar to mainstream medicine. Pre-disease conditions are "diagnosed" and "treated" with pharmaceuticals and other standard medical interventions as preventive measures to avoid the disease itself.

For example, high blood pressure has itself become a condition that is diagnosed, and blood pressure–lowering drugs, such as diuretics and beta blockers, are prescribed for the condition. Is high blood pressure a disease? Most people will probably think it is not, and typical cases of high blood pressure won't satisfy hybridism or normativism about disease (chapter 2). So blood pressure–lowering drugs are not usually targeting diseases. At least, interventions on cases of "primary prevention," which occur when a person has a risk factor for a disease but has not yet had the disease, involve targeting non-disease states. It is hard to see anything wrong with this practice in principle, and as noted above, a great amount of good can (in principle) be brought about by such preventive medical interventions. This suggests that the primary aims of medicine as suggested in the rest of this book—the curing of disease and the caring for the diseased—must be supplemented with the prevention of disease.

Alternatively, one could argue that standard medical practice should not be in the business of preventing disease. That would not be to say that disease prevention is not a prudential aim, only that mainstream medicine should not be the means to that end. Such a position, which is clearly at odds with contemporary medical practice, could be defended by noting how tiny the absolute effect sizes are for preventive medical interventions. Moreover, some critics note that the boundaries of the pre-disease states that medicine deems appropriate for intervening on have been creeping outward over time.

For example, the threshold for what counts as high blood pressure has been lowered over and over by the committees who are responsible for providing guidance on such matters (§6.2). Each time the threshold is lowered, many millions of additional people become categorizable as being in the pre-disease state that is an apt target for medical intervention—this phenomenon is sometimes called *disease creep*. This in turn leads to many millions of additional people being prescribed preventive medical interventions. Cynics note that the committees responsible for such decisions are composed of experts who have intricate financial conflicts of interest with the manufacturers of those preventive medical interventions.

There is a more general and less contingent question we can ask about preventive medicine. Preventive medicine aims to prevent the occurrence of disease. There are, in principle, uncountably many ways that we can achieve this. For example, seat belts can prevent bodily injury in a car crash. Dressing warmly in the winter can prevent one from catching the common cold. Deciding not to go skiing can prevent one from tearing a knee ligament. Properly consulting a mushroom field guide before cooking the mushrooms that you collected in the forest can prevent you from poisoning yourself. Most of us share the intuition, I reckon, that these preventive measures are not in the domain of medicine. So some practices of disease prevention are not in the domain of medicine. Are any? Many people answer yes. But if so, we are faced with a demarcation problem: some disease prevention practices are medical, and some are not. Figuring out which disease prevention practices are properly medical is not merely an academic concern, since it could turn out that much of contemporary medical practice falls on the non-medical side of this demarcation.

14.4 HEALTH INEQUALITIES

A health inequality is, quite simply, a disparity in health between individuals or groups. Consider a few examples: the life expectancy of people in Malawi is 47 years while in Japan it is 83 years, people from lower socioeconomic social strata have higher rates of type 2 diabetes than people from higher socioeconomic social strata, and children born into the poorest 20% of households are twice as likely to die by their fifth birthday as children born into the richest 20% of households. These differences are unlikely to be due to chance, but rather are probably due to political and economic circumstances, and because of this, health inequalities are typically said to be unfair—that is, the very concept of health inequality is associated with injustice.

The idea is that health inequalities are more than mere health differences that arise because of this or that cause. Health differences arise as a result of extrinsic chance (Jo slipped off his bicycle in the rain while Mary did not), intrinsic chance (Santiago has a growth hormone gene mutation while Hiroshi does not), or choice (Barsha eats well while Anastasiya does not). Health inequalities, on the other hand, arise as a result of social structures or relations that, broadly construed, are not merely unfair but are unjust (underemployed coal mining communities have higher rates of suicide than prosperous cities).

The work of social epidemiology, discussed in §14.2, is often employed to both discover the existence of health inequalities and to offer explanations for such inequalities. For instance, we saw that one of Michael Marmot's important findings is that higher social rank is correlated with better health, and he offers reasons to think that this is mediated via stress: people who have lower social rank have more stress at work, and this leads to worse health outcomes.

The main focus of concern regarding health inequalities, as Marmot's work suggests, has been inequalities between groups. Such groups can be defined by properties like socioeconomic class, gender, race, and nationality. When there are significant health inequalities between groups that are defined by such demographic properties, a reasonable assumption is that such differences do not arise by chance or by inevitable biological causes, but rather by contingent social features (such as access to resources). Since contingent social features can be changed with sufficient political will, many people hold the view that there is a prima facie argument in favor of doing so. Let's call this the *group viewpoint* of health inequalities, since the focus is on inequalities of health status between groups.

One issue that has attracted some debate is whether or not health differences between individuals can be deemed health inequalities. On the one hand, there can be significant health differences between individuals within a particular group, just as there are significant health differences between groups, and so, insofar as we are concerned with health inequalities generally, we ought to attend to health differences between individuals (let's call this the *individual viewpoint* of health inequality, since the view is concerned with health differences between individuals).

For example, suppose Ahmed, a middle-aged man who lives in London, has a heart attack at the age of sixty-three, and his neighbor Sumon does not. The individual viewpoint of health inequalities prompts us to ask not just about the particular causal or etiological details that differ between Ahmed and Sumon (perhaps Ahmed smokes, eats more meat, and has a higher body mass index than Sumon), because remember, the notion of a health inequality is characterized by a concern that health differences arise from unjust social structures. The individual viewpoint of health inequalities prompts us to ask if there is a difference between Ahmed's socioeconomic context and Sumon's socioeconomic context (perhaps Ahmed works as a low-paid security guard and Sumon works as a well-paid banker).

However, a problem with the individual viewpoint of health inequalities is that it is hard or impossible to know whether or not the causes of health differences between individuals are merely the result of those individuals' biological states, or choices that those individuals made throughout their lives, or chance, rather than contingent and politically modifiable features of their social context. Arguably this is an intractable epistemic problem, which serves to reaffirm the group viewpoint of health inequalities. This would not be to say that differences in health outcomes between individuals are not important, but only to say that there are two different kinds of differences: those that social planners can properly do something about and those that they cannot.

In response, the defender of the individual viewpoint could hold that differences between individuals are just as unfair as differences between groups, and moreover, the groups that motivate the group viewpoint are best thought of as convenient fictions for clumping individuals together—ultimately it is the health and health inequalities of individuals that matter.

From the perspective of social policy, one might hold that health inequalities that arise as a matter of individuals' choices (such as whether or not one exercises, smokes, or eats healthy food) are not unjust, and thus are not the sort of thing that public health or political interventions should be aiming to resolve. This is another consideration in favor of focusing on inequalities between groups. However, many health inequalities between individuals are not caused by those individuals' choices, but rather are caused by their social context or luck. Moreover, individuals' choices influence their group membership, and thus both health inequalities between individuals and health inequalities between groups can be influenced by the choices of individuals.

Emphasizing the importance of health inequalities between groups rather than individuals faces a problem with identifying the appropriate boundary with which to demarcate groups. The appearance of inequalities between groups is sensitive to how an overall population is subdivided into groups. This is another argument in favor of the individual viewpoint of health inequalities. On the other hand, individual health is difficult or impossible to measure, and beyond epistemic limitations, surely differences between individuals' health states are often due to chance and choice, and from a public policy perspective differences between individuals' health states are not the sorts of conditions that can readily be intervened on.

There are some groups for which boundaries can be identified in non-arbitrary ways, by reference to historical or political facts. For example, the aboriginal population of Canada is composed of the people whose ancestors were present in Canada before the arrival of European colonialists. Because of centuries of various forms of political oppression, the health of Canadian aboriginals is, on average, far worse than that of the non-aboriginal Canadian population. Canadian aboriginals suffer from respiratory diseases, for instance, at high rates, and this leads to acute care hospitalization rates which are higher than those of the non-aboriginal population. Social epidemiologists who study this argue that poor housing conditions, including crowded houses that need repairs and that have poor indoor air quality, contribute to the respiratory diseases of Canadian aboriginals.

Other groups that can be identified in non-arbitrary ways include citizens of particular nations. National boundaries create distinct socio-economic conditions. So, when we learn that the United States has an under-five childhood mortality rate of 6.5 per 1000 live births, and Estonia has an under-five mortality rate of 2.9, it is reasonable to ask why such a group-level health inequality exists: is there something unjust about the social or political context of the United States such that its childhood mortality rate is over double that of Estonia? (Now compare these under-five mortality rates to Angola, which has an under-five mortality rate of 157 per 1000 live births.)

FURTHER READING

Social epidemiology: McKeown (1976)
Preventive medicine: John (2011)
Health inequalities: Lewens (2010), Hausman (2007)

DISCUSSION QUESTIONS

1. Is the prevention paradox a real paradox?
2. What is the "McKeown thesis"? Is it compelling?

3. Are the ambitions of public health at odds with the ambitions of personalized medicine?
4. How should one draw the boundary around preventive interventions that are medical versus other sorts of preventive interventions?

REFERENCES

Alexandrova, Anna. 2018. "Can the science of well-being be objective?" *British Journal for the Philosophy of Science* 69 (2): 421–445.

Andersen, H. 2014. "A field guide to mechanisms: Part I." *Philosophy Compass* 9 (4): 274–283.

Biddle, Justin. 2007. "Lessons from the Vioxx debacle: What the privatization of science can teach us about social epistemology." *Social Epistemology* 21 (1): 21–39.

Biddle, Justin. 2013. "Institutionalizing dissent: A proposal for an adversarial system of pharmaceutical research." *Kennedy Institute of Ethics Journal* 23 (4): 325–353.

Biddle, Justin B. 2014. "Can patents prohibit research? On the social epistemology of patenting and licensing in science." *Studies in History and Philosophy of Science A* 45: 14–23.

Bluhm, Robyn, and Kirstin Borgerson. 2010. "Evidence-based medicine." In *Philosophy of Medicine*, edited by Fred Gifford, 203–237. Amsterdam: Elsevier.

Boorse, C. 1977. "Health as a theoretical concept." *Philosophy of Science* 44 (4): 542–573.

Boorse, C. 1997. "A rebuttal on health." In *What Is Disease?*, edited by J. Humber and R. Almeder, 1–134. Totowa, NJ: Humana.

Borgerson, K. 2005. "Evidence-based alternative medicine?" *Perspectives in Biology and Medicine* 48 (4): 502–515.

Bortolotti, Lisa. 2009. *Delusions and Other Irrational Beliefs*. Oxford: Oxford University Press.

Broadbent, Alex. 2009. "Causation and models of disease in epidemiology." *Studies in History and Philosophy of Biological and Biomedical Sciences* 40 (4): 302–311.

Brown, James. 2008. "Politics, method, and medical research." *Philosophy of Science* 75 (5): 756–766.

Brown, Matthew. 2013. "Value in science beyond underdetermination and inductive risk." *Philosophy of Science* 80: 829–839.

Carel, Havi. 2013. *Illness: The Cry of the Flesh*. London: Routledge.

Carel, H., and I. J. Kidd. 2014. "Epistemic injustice in healthcare: A philosophical analysis." *Medicine, Health Care and Philosophy* 17 (4): 529–540.

Carter, K. C. 2003. *The Rise of Causal Concepts of Disease*. Aldershot: Ashgate.

Cartwright, N. 2010. "What are randomised controlled trials good for?" *Philosophical Studies* 147: 59–70.

Cassell, E. J. 1991. *The Nature of Suffering and the Goals of Medicine*. New York: Oxford University Press.

Cassels, A. 2012. *Seeking Sickness: Medical Screening and the Misguided Hunt for Disease*. Vancouver: Greystone.

Clarke, B., D. Gillies, P. Illari, F. Russo, and J. Williamson. 2014. "Mechanisms and the evidence hierarchy." *Topoi* 33 (2): 339–360.

Cooper, Rachel. 2002. "Disease." *Studies in History and Philosophy of Biological and Biomedical Sciences* 33: 263–282.

Cooper, Rachel. 2004. "Why Hacking is wrong about human kinds." *British Journal for the Philosophy of Science* 55 (1): 73–85.

de Melo-Martin, Immaculada, and Kristen Intemann. 2011. "Feminist resources for biomedical research: Lessons from the HPV vaccines." *Hypatia* 26 (1): 79–101.

Douglas, Heather. 2000. "Inductive risk and values in science." *Philosophy of Science* 67 (4): 559–579.

Douglas, Heather. 2004. "The irreducible complexity of objectivity." *Synthese* 138: 453–473.

Elliott, Kevin C. 2011. "Direct and indirect roles for values in science." *Philosophy of Science* 78 (2): 303–324.

Engelhardt, H. Tristram. 1976. "Ideology and etiology." *Journal of Medicine and Philosophy* 1 (3): 256–268.

Ereshefsky, Marc. 2009. "Defining 'health' and 'disease.'" *Studies in History and Philosophy of Biological and Biomedical Sciences* 40: 221–227.

Fergusson, D., S. Doucette, K. C. Glass, S. Shapiro, D. Healy, P. Hebert, and B. Hutton. 2005. "Association between suicide attempts and selective serotonin reuptake inhibitors: Systematic review of randomised controlled trials." *BMJ* 330 (7488): 396.

Foucault, Michel. 1965. *Madness and Civilisation: A History of Insanity in the Age of Reason*. Translated by R. Howard. New York: Random House.

Fuller, J., and L. J. Flores. 2015. "The Risk GP Model: The standard model of prediction in medicine." *Studies in History and Philosophy of Biological and Biomedical Sciences* 54: 49–61.

Goldenberg, M. J., K. Borgerson, and R. Bluhm. 2009. "The nature of evidence in evidence-based medicine: Guest editors' introduction." *Perspectives in Biology and Medicine* 52 (2): 164–167.

Green, Sara, and Henrik Vogt. 2016. "Personalizing medicine: Disease prevention *in silico* and *in socio*." *Humana.Mente Journal of Philosophical Studies* 30: 105-145.

Gunnell, D., J. Saperia, and D. Ashby. 2005. "Selective serotonin reuptake inhibitors (SSRIs) and suicide in adults: meta-analysis of drug company data from placebo controlled, randomised controlled trials submitted to the MHRA's safety review." *BMJ* 330 (7488): 385.

Guyatt, G., et al. 1992. "Evidence-based medicine: A new approach to teaching the practice of medicine." *JAMA* 268 (17): 2420-2425.

Guyatt, G., and D. Rennie. 2001. *User's Guide to the Medical Literature.* Chicago: AMA Press.

Hacking, Ian. 1988. "Telepathy: Origins of randomisation in experimental design." *Isis* 79: 427-451.

Hacking, Ian. 1995. "The looping effects of human kinds." In *Causal Cognition*, edited by Dan Sperber, David Premack, and Ann James Premack, 351-383. Oxford: Clarendon.

Hacking, I. 2010. "Pathological withdrawl of refugee children seeking asylum in Sweden." *Studies in History and Philosophy of Biological and Biomedical Sciences* 41 (4): 309-317.

Hausman, Daniel. 2007. "What's wrong with health inequalities?" *Journal of Political Philosophy* 15 (1): 46-66.

Hausman, Daniel. 2015. *Valuing Health: Well-Being, Freedom, and Suffering.* New York: Oxford University Press.

Hesslow, Germund. 1993. "Do we need a concept of disease?" *Theoretical Medicine and Bioethics* 14: 1-14.

Hey, S. P., and A. S. Kesselheim. 2016. "Countering imprecision in precision medicine." *Science* 353 (6298): 448-449.

Holman, Bennett. 2015. "Why most sugar pills are not placebos." *Philosophy of Science* 82 (5): 1330-1343.

Holton, Richard, and Berridge, Kent. 2013. "Addiction between compulsion and choice." In *Addiction and Self-Control*, edited by Neil Levy, 239-268. Oxford: Oxford University Press.

Horwitz, Allan, and Jerome Wakefield. 2007. *Loss of Sadness: How Psychiatry Transformed Normal Sorrow into Depressive Disorder.* New York: Oxford University Press.

Howick, Jeremy. 2011a. "Exposing the vanities—and a qualified defense—of mechanistic reasoning in health care decision making." *Philosophy of Science* 78 (5): 926-940.

Howick, Jeremy. 2011b. *The Philosophy of Evidence-Based Medicine.* Oxford: Wiley-Blackwell.

Howick, Jeremy. 2017. "The relativity of 'placebos': Defending a modified version of Grünbaum's definition." *Synthese* 194 (4): 1363–1396.

Howson, Colin, and Peter Urbach. 1989. *Scientific Reasoning: The Bayesian Approach*. La Salle, IL: Open Court.

Illari, Phyllis McKay. 2011. "Mechanistic evidence: Disambiguating the Russo–Williamson thesis." *International Studies in the Philosophy of Science* 25 (2): 139–157.

Illich, Ivan. 1975. *Medical Nemesis: The Expropriation of Health*. London: Marion Boyars.

Ioannidis, J. P. 2005. "Why most published research findings are false." *PLoS Med* 2 (8): e124.

Ioannidis, J. P. 2011. "An epidemic of false claims: Competition and conflicts of interest distort too many medical findings." *Scientific American* 304 (6): 16.

John, Stephen. 2011. "Expert testimony and epistemological free-riding: The MMR controversy." *Philosophical Quarterly* 61 (244): 496–517.

John, Stephen D. 2013. "Cancer screening, risk stratification and the ethics of apt categorisation: A case study." In *Ethics in Public Health and Health Policy: Concepts, Methods, Case Studies*, edited by D. Strech, I. Hirschberg, and G. Marckmann, 141–152. Dordrecht: Springer Netherlands.

Jukola, Saana. 2015. "Meta-analysis, ideals of objectivity, and the reliability of medical knowledge." *Science and Technology Studies* 28(3): 101–120.

Kendler, Kenneth S., and Josef Parnas, eds. 2012. *Philosophical Issues in Psychiatry II: Nosology*. Oxford: Oxford University Press.

Kennedy, A. G. 2016. "Evaluating diagnostic tests." *Journal of Evaluation in Clinical Practice* 22 (4): 575–579.

Khalidi, M. 2013. *Natural Categories and Human Kinds*. Cambridge: Cambridge University Press.

Kingma, Elselijn. 2007. "What is it to be healthy?" *Analysis* 67 (294): 128–133.

Kitcher, Philip. 2001. *Science, Truth, and Democracy*. Oxford: Oxford University Press.

Krimsky, S. 2003. *Science in the Private Interest*. Lanham, MD: Rowman and Littlefield.

Kuorikoski, Jaakko, and Samuli Pöyhönen. 2012. "Looping kinds and social mechanisms." *Sociological Theory* 30 (3): 187–205.

LaFollette, Hugh, and Niall Shanks. 1996. *Brute Science: Dilemmas of Animal Experimentation*. London: Routledge.

Lange, M. 2007. "The end of diseases." *Philosophical Topics* 35 (1/2): 265–292.

Leibovici, Leonard. 2001. "Effects of remote, retroactive intercessory prayer on outcomes in patients with bloodstream infection: Randomised controlled trial." *BMJ* 323 (7327): 1450–1451.

Lemoine, M. 2013. "Defining disease beyond conceptual analysis: An analysis of conceptual analysis in philosophy of medicine." *Theoretical Medicine and Bioethics* 34 (4): 309–325.

Leuridan, Bert, and Erik Weber. 2011. "The IARC and mechanistic evidence." In *Causality in the Sciences*, edited by P. Illari, F. Russo, and J. Williamson, 91–109. New York: Oxford University Press.

Lewens, T. 2010. "What are 'natural inequalities'?" *Philosophical Quarterly* 60 (239): 264–285.

Longino, Helen. 1990. *Science as Social Knowledge: Values and Objectivity in Scientific Inquiry* Princeton: Princeton University Press.

Marmot, Michael. 2004. *Status Syndrome: How Your Social Standing Directly Affects Your Health and Life Expectancy.* London: Bloomsbury.

Marquis, Don. 1989. "Why abortion is immoral." *Journal of Philosophy* 86 (4): 183–202.

Mayo, Deborah. 1996. *Error and the Growth of Experimental Knowledge.* Chicago: University of Chicago Press.

McClimans, Leah. 2013. "The role of measurement in establishing evidence." *Journal of Medicine and Philosophy* 38 (5): 520–538.

McKeown, Thomas. 1976. *The Modern Rise of Population.* London: Edward Arnold.

McMahan, J. 1995. "The metaphysics of brain death." *Bioethics* 9 (2): 91–126.

McMahan, J. 2002. *The Ethics of Killing: Problems at the Margins of Life.* New York: Oxford University Press.

Miller, Boaz. 2013. "When is consensus knowledge based? Distinguishing shared knowledge from mere agreement." *Synthese* 190 (7): 1293–1316.

Moynihan, Ray, Iona Heath, and David Henry. 2002. "Selling sickness: The pharmaceutical industry and disease mongering." *BMJ* 324 (7342): 886–891.

Murphy, Dominic. 2006. *Psychiatry in the Scientific Image.* Cambridge, MA: MIT Press.

Murphy, D. 2010. "Explanation in psychiatry." *Philosophy Compass* 5 (7): 602–610.

Nagel, T. 1970. "Death." *Noûs* 4 (1): 73–80.

Nordenfeldt, Lennart. 1987. *On the Nature of Health: An Action-Theoretic Approach.* Dordrecht: Reidel.

Parrott, Matthew. 2016. "Bayesian models, delusional beliefs, and epistemic possibilities." *British Journal for the Philosophy of Science* 67 (1): 271–296.

Pickard, H. 2015. "Psychopathology and the ability to do otherwise." *Philosophy and Phenomenological Research* 90 (1): 135–163.

Pinto, M. F. 2015. "Commercialization and the limits of well-ordered science." *Perspectives on Science* 23 (2): 173–191.

Plutynski, A. 2012. "Ethical issues in cancer screening and prevention." *Journal of Medicine and Philosophy* 37 (3): 310–323.

Plutynski, Anya. 2017. "Safe, or sorry? Cancer screening and inductive risk." In *Exploring Inductive Risk*, edited by Kevin Elliott and Ted Richards, 149–169. Oxford: Oxford University Press.

President's Commission. 1981. "Guidelines for the determination of death." *JAMA* 246 (19): 2184–2186.

Ratcliffe, Matthew. 2010. "Depression, guilt, and emotional depth." *Inquiry* 53 (6): 602–626.

Rawlins, Michael. 2008. "*De testimonio*: On the evidence for decisions about the use of therapeutic interventions." *Clinical Medicine* 8: 579–588.

Resnik, David. 2007. *The Price of Truth: How Money Affects the Norms of Science*. New York: Oxford University Press.

Sackett, David L. 1979. "Bias in analytic research." *Journal of Chronic Diseases* 32 (1–2): 51–63.

Salmon, W. 1997. *Causality and Explanation*. New York: Oxford University Press.

Schaffner, K. F. 2006. "Reduction: The Cheshire cat problem and a return to roots." *Synthese* 151 (3): 377–402.

Simon, Jeremy. 2010 "Playing the odds: A new response to Lucretius's symmetry argument." *European Journal of Philosophy* 18 (3): 414–424.

Singer, Peter. 1994. *Rethinking Life and Death: The Collapse of Our Traditional Ethics*. Melbourne: Text.

Sober, Elliott. 2008. *Evidence and Evolution: The Logic Behind the Science*. Cambridge: Cambridge University Press.

Solomon, Miriam. 2001. *Social Empiricism*. Cambridge, MA: MIT Press.

Solomon, Miriam. 2011. "Group judgment and the medical consensus conference." In *Philosophy of Medicine*, edited by Fred Gifford, 239–254. Amsterdam: Elsevier.

Solomon, Miriam. 2015. *Making Medical Knowledge*. Oxford: Oxford University Press.

Sprenger, Jan. 2016. "Bayesianism vs. frequentism in statistical inference." In *Oxford Handbook of Probability and Philosophy*, edited by A. Hájek and C. Hitchcock. Oxford: Oxford University Press.

Steel, Daniel. 2007. *Across the Boundaries*. Oxford: Oxford University Press.

Stegenga, Jacob. 2011. "Is meta-analysis the platinum standard?" *Studies in History and Philosophy of Biological and Biomedical Sciences* 42: 497-507.

Stegenga, Jacob. 2015a. "Measuring effectiveness." *Studies in the History and Philosophy of Biological and Biomedical Sciences* 54: 62-71.

Stegenga, J. 2015b. "Effectiveness of medical interventions." *Studies in the History and Philosophy of Biological and Biomedical Sciences* 54: 34-44.

Stegenga, Jacob. 2017. "Drug regulation and the inductive risk calculus." In *Exploring Inductive Risk*, edited by Ted Richards and Kevin Elliott, 17-36. Oxford: Oxford University Press.

Stegenga, Jacob. 2018. *Medical Nihilism*. Oxford: Oxford University Press.

Sullivan, Jacqueline A. 2010. "Reconsidering 'spatial memory' and the Morris water maze." *Synthese* 177 (2): 261-283.

Tabb, K. 2015. "Psychiatric progress and the assumption of diagnostic discrimination." *Philosophy of Science* 82 (5): 1047-1058.

Teira, David. 2017. "Testing oncological treatments in the era of personalized medicine." In *Philosophy of Molecular Medicine*, edited by G. Boniolo and M. Nathan, 236-251. London: Routledge.

Tekin, Serife. 2014. "The missing self in Hacking's looping effects." In *Classifying Psychopathology: Mental Kinds and Natural Kinds*, edited by H. Kincaid and J. A. Sullivan, 227-256. Cambridge, MA: MIT Press.

Thompson, Judith. 1971. "A defence of abortion." *Philosophy and Public Affairs* 1 (1): 47-66.

Tonelli, Mark. 2006. "Integrating evidence into clinical practice: an alternative to evidence-based approaches." *Journal of Evaluation in Clinical Practice* 12 (3): 248-256.

Tsou, Jonathan Y. 2007. "Hacking on the looping effects of psychiatric classifications: What is an interactive and indifferent kind?" *International Studies in the Philosophy of Science* 21 (3): 329-344.

Tsou, Jonathan Y. 2011. "The importance of history for philosophy of psychiatry: The case of the *DSM* and psychiatric classification." *Journal of the Philosophy of History* 5 (3): 446-470.

Tulodziecki, Dana. 2013. "Shattering the myth of Semmelweis." *Philosophy of Science* 80 (5): 1065-1075.

Upshur, Ross. 2002. "If not evidence, then what? Or does medicine really need a base?" *Journal of Evaluation in Clinical Practice* 8 (2): 113-119.

Urbach, P. 1985. "Randomization and the design of experiments." *Philosophy of Science* 52 (2): 256-273.

Weber, Marcel. 2005. *Philosophy of Experimental Biology*. Cambridge: Cambridge University Press.

Wilholt, Torsten. 2009. "Bias and values in scientific research." *Studies in History and Philosophy of Science A* 40 (1): 92–101.

Williams, Bernard. 1973. *Problems of the Self*. Cambridge: Cambridge University Press.

Wootton, D. 2006. *Bad Medicine: Doctors Doing Harm since Hippocrates.* New York: Oxford University Press.

Worrall, John. 2002. "What evidence in evidence-based medicine?" *Philosophy of Science* 69: S316–S330.

flibanserin, 84

food poisoning, 96

Foucault, Michel, 198

free will, 96

frequentism, 126, 138, 141, 151, 154–56,
   219–20

Freudian theory, 129, 192

Fromm, Erich, 200

fugue, 93

function, 11, 23–25

Galen, 62

Galileo, 215

generalized anxiety disorder, 78

genome-wide association study, 65,
   195

germ theory, 73, 75, 143, 163, 196

gunshot wound, 91

Hacking, Ian, 88–89, 92–94

heart attack, 85, 86, 164, 165, 227–28,
   231

heart disease, 57, 63, 164, 208, 211

Hegel, G. W. F., 213

Herceptin. *See* trastuzumab

Hesslow, Germund, 32–33

Hill, Bradford, 121, 136, 142–43, 146–47

Hill criteria. *See* Hill, Bradford

Hippocrates, 162

HIV, 53, 186

holistic medicine. *See* alternative
   medicine

Holmes, Oliver Wendell, Sr., 163

homeopathy, 2, 159, 166–67, 169

hormone-replacement therapy, 122

human kinds, 88–89

humoral theory, 62, 122

Huntington's disease, 178

hwabyeong, 80, 89, 90–91

hydrotherapy, 197

hygienists, 69

hypertension, 21, 29, 85–86, 228–29

idiopathic diseases, 177

imipramine, 198

incremental cost-effectiveness ratio
   (ICER), 226

inductive risk, 131–34, 176, 185, 220

infectious disease: discovery, 143–44;
   eradication, 91; monocausal model
   of disease, 51, 57, 63; nosology, 58,
   60; research priorities, 211, 215;
   treatment, 75, 215, 222

inference to the best explanation, 3,
   175, 177

influenza, 176, 194

insulin, 10–11, 23, 54, 59, 75, 110, 161,
   162, 173, 215

intellectual property, 2, 128, 207, 212–
   16, 219

INUS theory of causation, 53, 56–57

Ioannidis, John, 163

iproniazid, 198

ivacaftor, 65

Kendler, Kenneth, 88

Khrushchev, Nikita, 199

Kitcher, Philip, 211–12

Koch, Robert. *See* Koch's postulates

Koch's postulates, 54, 143–44

koro, 80

Kuhn, Thomas, 202

Laing, R. D., 198

Leibovici study. *See* retroactive intercessory prayer

leprosy, 98

libertarianism about medical research,
   209–12

Lind, James, 122